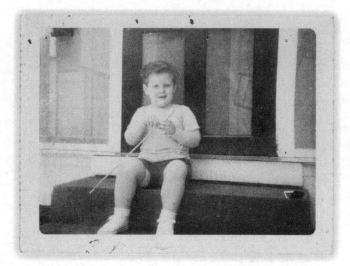

The
Elephant
in the
Room

One Fat Man's Quest
to Get Smaller
in a Growing
America

Tommy
Tomlinson

Simon & Schuster

New York   London   Toronto   Sydney   New Delhi

Simon & Schuster
1230 Avenue of the Americas
New York, NY 10020

First Simon & Schuster hardcover edition January 2019

SIMON & SCHUSTER and colophon are registered
trademarks of Simon & Schuster, Inc.

For information about special discounts for bulk purchases,
please contact Simon & Schuster Special Sales at
1-866-506-1949 or business@simonandschuster.com.

The Simon & Schuster Speakers Bureau can bring authors to your live event.
For more information or to book an event, contact the
Simon & Schuster Speakers Bureau at 1-866-248-3049 or
visit our website at www.simonspeakers.com.

Interior design by Ruth Lee-Mui

Manufactured in the United States of America

1   3   5   7   9   10   8   6   4   2

Library of Congress Cataloging-in-Publication Data is available.

ISBN 978-1-5011-1161-7
ISBN 978-1-5011-1163-1 (ebook)

For Alix

Contents

CONTENTS

It's quite a mystery, albeit largely unacknowledged, to be alive, and, quite simply, in order to remain alive you must keep eating. My notion, scarcely original, is that if you eat badly you are very probably living badly.

—Jim Harrison

So come on, fatso, and just bust a move.

—Young MC

KILLING THE HOG

I have this dream. We're on a road trip, out in this house in the country, and I'm trying to talk to my wife. But this hog gets in the house. It stinks and it's slick to the touch and I can't keep it off me. I push it away but it keeps plowing back and I see tusks. I finally shove it out the door. Now I'm in bed. Here comes the hog again. I can barely stave it off with my hands. It's all over me. I get to my feet and kick it and ram it with my shoulder and we tumble out into the yard. My mouth is coated with hog-slime, and I reach in and scrape it off my tongue. I'm half-dressed, stinking, miserable. Suddenly we're back in a room and I can sense I'm being watched. Three or four official-looking people are lined up at a table, like judges on a panel. One of them says, "Here's what you have to do."

I wake up knowing two things.

One, I have to kill the hog.

Two, the hog is a part of me.

NEW YEAR'S EVE, 2014

I weigh 460 pounds.

Those are the hardest words I've ever had to write. Nobody knows that number—not my wife, not my doctor, not my closest friends. It feels like confessing a crime. The average American male weighs 195 pounds; I'm two of those guys, with a ten-year-old left over. I'm the biggest human being most people who know me have ever met, or ever will.

The government definition of obesity is a body mass index of thirty or more. My BMI is 60.7. My shirts are size XXXXXXL, which the big-and-tall stores shorten to 6X. I'm six-foot-one, or seventy-three inches tall. My waist is sixty inches around. I'm nearly a sphere.

Those are the numbers. This is how it feels.

I'm on the subway in New York City, standing in the aisle, clinging to the pole. I live in Charlotte and don't visit New York much, so I don't have a feel for how subway cars move. I'm praying this one doesn't lurch around a corner or slam to a stop because I'm terrified of falling. Part of it is embarrassment. When a fat guy falls, it's hard to get up. But what really scares me is the chance I might land on somebody. I glance at the people wedged around me. None of them could take my weight. It would be an avalanche. Some of them stare at me and I figure they're thinking the same thing. There's an old woman sitting three feet away. One slip and I'd crush her. I grip the pole harder. My palms start to sweat and all of a sudden I flash back—

to elementary school in Georgia, standing in the aisle on the bus. The driver hollers at me to find a seat. He can't take us home until everybody sits down. I'm the only one standing. Every time I spot an open space, somebody slides to the edge of the seat and covers it up. Nobody wants the fat boy mashed in next to them. I freeze, helpless. The driver glares at me in the rearview mirror. An older kid sitting in front of me—a redhead, freckles, I'll never forget his face—has a cast on his right arm. He reaches back and starts clubbing me with it, below the waist, out of the driver's line of sight. He catches me in the groin and it hurts, but not as much as the shame when the other kids laugh and the bus driver gets up and storms toward me—

and the train stops and jolts me back into now.

I peel my hands from the pole and get off. I climb the stairs to the street and step to the side to catch my breath. I'm wheezing like a thirty-year smoker. My legs wobble from the climb. I'm meeting a friend near Central Park at a place called the Brooklyn Diner. Why is there a Brooklyn Diner in Manhattan? Are Manhattan diners not up to lofty Brooklyn standards? I have time to think about such things. I'm fifteen minutes early, on purpose, because I have to find a safe place to sit.

The night before, I had Googled "Brooklyn Diner interior" to get an idea of the layout. Now I scan the space like a gangster, looking for danger spots. The booths are too small—I can't squeeze in. The bar stools are bolted to the floor—they're too close to the bar and my ass would hang off the back. I check the tables, gauging the chairs. Flimsy chairs creak and quake beneath me. These look solid. I spot a table in the corner with just enough room. I sit down slowly—the chair seems OK, yep, it'll hold me up. For the first time in an hour, I take an untroubled breath.

My friend shows up on time. By then I've scouted out the menu. Eggs, bacon, toast, coffee. A few bites and the shame fades. At least for a little while.

By any reasonable standard, I have won life's lottery. I grew up with two loving parents in a peaceful house. I've spent my whole career doing work that thrills me—writing for newspapers and magazines. I married the best woman I've ever known, Alix Felsing, and I love her more now than when my heart first tumbled for her. We live in an old house in Charlotte with a yellow Lab mutt named Fred. We're blessed with strong families and a deep bench of friends. Our lives are full of music and laughter. I wouldn't swap with anyone.

Except on those mornings when I wake up and take a long naked look in the mirror.

My body is a car wreck. Skin tags—long, mole-like growths caused by chafing—dangle under my arms and down in my crotch. I have breasts where my chest ought to be. My belly is strafed with more stretch marks than a mother of five. My stomach hangs below my waist, giving me what the Urban Dictionary calls a front butt— as if some twisted Dr. Frankenstein grafted an extra rear end on the wrong side. Varicose veins bulge from my thighs. My calves and shins are rust-colored and shiny from a condition called chronic venous insufficiency. (You never want any medical condition that contains the words *chronic* and *insufficiency*.) Here's what it means:

The veins in my legs aren't strong enough to push all the blood back up toward my heart, so it pools in my capillaries and forces little dots of iron up under my skin. The veins are failing because of the pressure caused by 460 pounds pushing downward with every step I take. My body is crumbling under its own gravity.

Some days, when I see that disaster staring back, I get so mad that I pound my gut with my fists, as if I could beat the fat out of me. Other times the sight sinks me into a blue fog that can ruin an hour or a morning or a day. But most of the time what I feel is sadness over how much life I've wasted. When I was a kid, I never climbed a tree or learned to swim. When I was in my twenties, I never took a girl home from a bar. Now I'm fifty, and I've never hiked a mountain or ridden a skateboard or done a cartwheel. I've missed out on so many adventures, so many good times, because I was too fat to try. Sometimes, when I could've tried anyway, I didn't have the guts. I've done a lot of things I'm proud of. But I've never believed I could do anything truly great, because I've failed so many times at the one crucial challenge in my life.

What the hell is wrong with me?

What the hell is wrong with *us*?

As I write this, the Centers for Disease Control estimates that seventy-nine million American adults—forty percent of women, and thirty-five percent of men—qualify as obese. That's more than the total attendance of every Major League Baseball game last year. Our kids are right behind us—the obesity rate among American children is seventeen percent and climbing. Our collective waistline laps over every boundary—age, race, gender, politics, culture. In our fractured country, we all agree on one thing: second helpings.

Fat America runs on the fuel of easy and cheap junk food, motivated by constant ads for burgers and beer, soothed and sated by oversized portions. At most movie theaters now, a small soft drink is thirty-two ounces. No reasonable definition of *small* encompasses a quart of Coke. The English language, like my elastic-waisted cargo shorts, has stretched to fit our expanding country.

As every fat person knows, there's no such thing as a cheap buffet—you always pay later, one way or another. Fat America comes with a devastating bill. According to government estimates, Americans pay $147 billion a year in medical costs related to obesity. That's roughly equal to the entire budget for the U.S. army. But the money is just part of the cost. Every fat person, and every fat person's family, pays with anger and heartache and pain. For every one of us who can't shed the weight, there are spouses and parents and kids and friends who grieve for us. We carve lines in their faces. We sentence them to long years alone.

I know this from experience. I also feel it like a burning knife right now. Because my sister, Brenda Williams, died on Christmas Eve.

One of the great joys in our family was getting Brenda to laugh. If somebody cracked an off-color joke, her eyes cranked open wide and her eyebrows flew up her forehead like a cartoon. Sometimes she let out a low cackle that tickled me even more. She and her husband, Ed Williams, had been married forty-three years and raised three kids. Brenda was never happier than when she had a houseful of the people she loved. But she didn't laugh as much the last few years. Her weight scared her and isolated her and eventually it killed her.

Brenda was sixty-three and weighed well north of two hundred pounds. Her feet swelled so much she could hardly wear shoes. Her thighs cramped so bad, with so little warning, that she was afraid to drive. For years she dealt with sores on her legs caused by the swelling. They leaked fluid and wouldn't heal. In late December, one of the sores got infected. Brenda was tough, so by the time she admitted she was sick, she was in deep trouble. Her husband took her to the emergency room in Jesup, Georgia, as we were heading to Tennessee to spend Christmas with Alix's folks. My brother called at two in the morning on Christmas Eve and said things were getting worse. We tried to sleep for a couple of hours, got up, and got on the road. The infection turned out to be MRSA. It spread so goddamn fast. We were somewhere outside Asheville when my brother sent a text: *She's gone.*

The funeral was on my mom's eighty-second birthday. She cried tears from the bottom of the ocean. She lived next door to Brenda and Ed for almost twenty years—we moved her there after she retired. She spent so many nights telling stories around Brenda and Ed's dining-room table. Now she won't go back in their house. All she can see is the empty space where Brenda used to be. The infection was the official cause of Brenda's death, but her weight killed her, sure as poison.

What happens when someone close to you dies? People bring food.

It arrived at Brenda and Ed's house, and my mom's, within minutes and in great quantities. Neighbors made potato salad and pecan pie. Folks who didn't cook brought cold cuts and light bread. One of Ed's friends arranged for the Western Sizzlin down the road to send a whole rolling cart of meat and vegetables. No matter where you stood, you were no more than ten feet from fried chicken. I crammed everything I could onto my double-thick paper plate. The sugar and grease pushed back the grief, just for a minute or two, long enough to breathe.

This is the terrible catch-22. The thing that soothes the pain prolongs it. The thing that brings me back to life pushes me closer to the grave.

I think a lot these days about a guy named David Poole. David and I worked together at the *Charlotte Observer*—he was a brilliant NASCAR writer when I was the local columnist. I weighed more than David, but he was shorter and rounder. We didn't look alike, but we were two fat guys with our pictures in the paper, so readers lumped us together. People would come up to me on the street and ask if I was him. He was one of the smartest guys I've ever met, a great reporter with a fearless voice, one of Alix's closest friends for years. David died of a heart attack when he was fifty. I'm about to turn fifty-one.

Guys like us don't make it to sixty.

Some of us rot away from diabetes or blow out an artery from high blood pressure, but a heart attack is what I worry about most. My doctor likes to quote a statistic: In a third of the cases of heart disease, the first symptom is death. Right now my heart tests out fine. But I can hear it thumping in my temples, eighty-some beats a minute even when I'm resting, and I know I make it work too hard. Sometimes, when it's quiet in the house, I close my eyes and listen to it strain, praying that it won't just stop like a needle lifted off a record. Every day I wonder if this is the day I might keel over in my office chair or at the bookstore or (God help me) at the wheel of my car. At 460 pounds, I'm lucky to have made it this far. It's like holding twenty at the blackjack table and waving at the dealer for another card. Without a miracle, I'm bound to bust.

Bless me, Father, for I have sinned: I lust after greasy double cheeseburgers and fried chicken legs and Ruffles straight out of the bag. I covet hot Krispy Kreme doughnuts that melt on my tongue. I worship bowls full of peanut M&M's, first savoring them one by one, then stuffing my mouth with handfuls, then wetting my finger to pick up those last bits of chocolate dust and candy shell. My brain pings with pleasure; my taste buds groan with desire. This happens over and over, day after day, and that is how I got here, closer to the end of my life than the beginning, weighing almost a quarter of a ton.

More than anything, I want to buy time. I want to write every story that needs to come out of me. I want to be the old retired guy with nothing to do but read books and play cards. I want to pack a bag and fill a cooler and get in the car and just ramble. I want to kiss Alix on her eightieth birthday, and I want her to kiss me on mine. I want to look back and be able to say with an honest heart that my years were not wasted.

I can't say that now. I have wasted so many.

After we got back from Georgia, I hung my black suit in the

closet. It's my only suit. I bought it seventeen years ago to get married in. I had to have it cut special at a big men's store called Thick and Thin. We ended up going with a tuxedo for the wedding, but I kept the suit. Sometimes it's a little tight, sometimes a little loose, but it more or less fits because I've been more or less the same size all these years. I've worn it to other people's weddings, to a few fancy parties, to a couple of anniversary dinners. Mostly I've worn it to funerals. I wore it to Brenda's. Before long, I fear, it's the suit I will be buried in.

There are radical options for people like me. There are boot camps where I could spend thousands of dollars to have trainers whip me into shape. There are crash diets and medications with dangerous side effects. And, of course, there is weight-loss surgery. Several people I know have done it. Some say it saved them. Others had life-threatening complications. A few are just as miserable as they were before. I don't judge any people who try to find their own way. I speak only for myself here: For me, surgery feels like giving up. I know that the first step of twelve-step programs is admitting that you're powerless over your addiction. But I don't feel powerless yet. The hog in my dream terrifies me. He's vicious and strong. But somewhere under all these folds of fat is a small part of me that still believes I can take him.

Being a journalist, I work best on deadline. Do you know where the word comes from? In the Civil War, in my home state of Georgia, there was a horrible Confederate prison called Andersonville. Tens of thousands of captured Union soldiers starved and suffered there. More than thirteen thousand died. Inside the prison, there was a wooden railing that separated the prisoners from the stockade walls. It wasn't much of a barrier—except that when any prisoners tried to climb it, or even touch it, the guards shot them on sight. That railing was the deadline.

In my life I am the prisoner, and I am the guard. With every big meal, and every day spent on the couch, I have reached closer to the railing, and I have fired a slow bullet aimed for my heart.

Here is my deadline. By the end of 2015, one year from now, I am going to lose weight and get in shape. I'm not going to set a number, because every time I've done that, I've fallen short. My goal is to prove that I can head down the right path and stay on it. I have to show that I won't quit even when it's hard, because it's going to be hard.

If I get to the end of the year and I've failed, every option goes back on the table: boot camp, pills, surgery, everything.

I have a long history of doing this the wrong way. I've thought about a few simple things that might help me do it right. But it will take more than just a meal plan and a walk every morning. I have to dig deep.

One weekend in college, I went to Atlanta to visit Virgil Ryals and Perry Beard, my two closest friends, who at the time were students at Georgia Tech. They had a bunch of people over to their apartment, and everybody was drinking, and somebody started up a game called Questions. One person starts off by asking anybody else in the group a question. That person doesn't answer the question; instead, he or she immediately turns to somebody else and asks a different question. You go until somebody can't think of a question. It's harder than it sounds. Especially if you've been pounding Jose Cuervo and Bud Lights.

A couple of guys I didn't know were at the party. They were drunker than everybody else, but they had come up with a winning strategy. Every time one of them had to take a turn, he'd look at me and go: "Tommy, why are you so fat?"

They thought this was hilarious. It was even funnier, to them, that I kept losing the game—once they asked me that, I couldn't stammer out a question to anybody else. After three or four rounds of this, I slipped off into the kitchen. I thought about going back in with my own question: *How would you like me to beat the shit out of you?* My fists were ready, but my heart wasn't in it. Those guys were assholes, but they were asking the same question I had asked myself my whole life.

Why am I so fat?

I've never really understood why I eat so much and why I've never been able to slow down for good. I need to make sense of how I grew up, crack the shell on some old memories, reach down and feel around in dark places, find out what is waiting down there in the mud.

I fight my cravings every day. My weight affects everything I do. It's going to kill me if I don't change.

I've spent a lifetime telling other people's stories. My weight is the biggest story of my life, but I haven't told it—because I was embarrassed, because I was afraid, because I knew I didn't understand myself.

It's time to tell it. It's time to go to work.

I'm on deadline.

One

A CHOCOLATE MILK
CARTON OF LOVE

The slice of cheese is the color of the sun. I'm three or four years old, alone in the dirt yard of our little house on St. Simons Island, down on the Georgia coast, halfway between Savannah and Jacksonville. My mom is watching me through the kitchen window. Next door is a kindergarten called Alice's Wonderland. Some older kids are over there playing kickball. They won't pay me any attention. So I go inside and open the fridge and grab a slice of individually wrapped processed American cheese—waxy and square, yellow and orange, perfect and beautiful. I unwrap it and fold it into quarters so it will pass through the chain-link fence. I go back outside and now the kids notice me. A couple of them come over and take the pieces. One of them throws me the ball. We kick it back and forth over the fence until they have to go inside. Then I go back in to get a slice of my own.

From then on I knew: Food is connection, food is friendship, food is a certain kind of love.

There's a photo of me from around that time. I look about the same now as I did back then. Same Shoney's Big Boy haircut. Same belly stretching my white T-shirt. Same thighs too big for my shorts. At birth I was normal-sized—seven pounds, one ounce. But by the time I was old enough to know anything, I was fat. I've never been not fat.

We lived four blocks from the ocean in a house with a char-treuse fiberglass awning and a palm tree in the yard. Those years come back to me in smells. The salty funk of the breeze coming off the marsh. The rotten-egg stench of the pulp mills from over on the mainland in Brunswick. The DDT from the mosquito truck that rode down our street at dusk, blowing clouds of bug poison from a nozzle in the truck bed.

And, most of all, the aroma of catfish frying in our kitchen. You could hand me a bushel of honeysuckle and it wouldn't smell as sweet as that grease in my mama's cast-iron pan.

Rich people have always lived on St. Simons—it was once one of the largest cotton plantations in the country—and tourists come for a taste of salt water and Spanish moss. But in the early sixties a working man and woman could find a little wafer of land there and start themselves a life. That's what my mom and dad did. They met on the job at SeaPak, a seafood processing plant on the is-land. My mom, Virginia, supervised one of the packing lines. My dad, L.M., fixed and maintained the big machines. When they got married in 1963, my dad had a cast on his left hand from getting his fingers mangled at work. When I was born, on January 4, 1964, the mortgage payment for our house was fifty dollars a month. We had a weary Pontiac station wagon and a VW Bug with holes in the floorboard. Nobody used the phrase *working poor* back then. But that's what we were.

My dad wore blue work shirts with his name patched on the chest. He always looked a little caved-in, as if somebody had just thrown him a sandbag, and his shoulders were sloped instead of squared. But his forearms were creased with muscle, and when I hugged him, his back felt like an oak. He was built for work, not for show. He had a bald spot the whole time I knew him, and held his comb-over down with a greasy gel called Score. It smelled like spilled gasoline. I put it in my hair for years so I could be like him.

Old age has shrunk my mama some. I used to rest my chin on her head when I hugged her, and now I have to bend down to do it. I remember her with big hair and big glasses and sweat beading on her upper lip as she cooked supper or pulled weeds. She wouldn't go to the movies because they wouldn't let her smoke. Even now, on the back side of eighty, tethered to an oxygen hose, she is as tough as boat rope.

They had it about as hard as white people could have it in the first part of the twentieth century. They were born into Depression families of South Georgia sharecroppers, picking cotton on somebody else's land. They bent over in the sun all day until the backs of their necks blistered—that's where the word *redneck* comes from. Every day but Sunday, from the time they could walk, my people spent all day in the heat, dragging cotton sacks that got heavier with every row. Their fingers bled from the thorny seedpods under the cotton boll. Mama's brother, my uncle Junior, would start fights with his brothers to get out of the field. If that didn't work, he would stand on a stump and holler at God to send rain.

The men who owned the fields deducted the cost of every last seed and broken hoe handle. When it came time to settle up, the sharecroppers' share vanished from the books. My mama's family moved from shack to shack, one step ahead of the rent. My aunt Mae remembers the nicest place they ever lived being the one that didn't need pasteboard to cover the cracks in the walls. The seven kids bathed in the same water, one after another, in a washtub. They got one pair of shoes a year and an orange at Christmas.

My dad was seventeen years older. The times he grew up in were even worse. He didn't like to talk about it.

I never knew my grandfather—my mother's father—but he was a one-man country song. One year he took the family's payout from the cotton harvest, bought a car, drove it to Florida, and totaled it. He worked for a time as a cop, and later did time in prison for shooting a woman. My grandmother raised the kids mostly by herself. But when she was still a young woman, she had a stroke and lost the use of her left side. My mom was the oldest girl still living at home. So at age twelve, she took over the household.

The main job was keeping the family fed. Every morning she got up before light and made two or three pans of biscuits on the woodstove. She mixed some extra flour with bacon drippings for white gravy. That was breakfast. Then she'd pour water over black-eyed peas or lima beans and leave them to simmer while everybody went out to the fields. Those beans and cornbread were lunch and supper. If they were lucky, there was a hunk of ham to throw in the pot. Once in a great while they had a few chickens running around. One day, when she was little, Mama had to kill a chicken for supper. She wrung its neck and it broke her heart. She has refused to eat chicken ever since.

In every picture of my family from back then, the men and women are as lean and strong as deer. They didn't have to diet. They had never heard of a gym. Their lives were exercise. When they weren't picking cotton, they chopped wood for the stove or hauled water from the well. They had the stamina of triathletes. They shoveled in all the food they had just to keep them going. They could down half a dozen biscuits without an ounce of regret. Their eating habits landed hard in my DNA. Turns out you don't burn off those biscuits so fast when you work at a desk in air-conditioning.

My mom had two kids from her first marriage—Brenda and my brother, Ronald Bennett. They were a lot older than me—out on their own by the time I was old enough to remember. I was my dad's only child. He was forty-eight when I was born. He had waited a long time to be a father. He spoiled me as much as he could with the money they had. When I started to show an interest in basketball, he built me a goal out of plywood and plumbing pipe. He bought me the special G.I. Joes with the Kung Fu Grip even though he just about passed out when he saw how much they cost. I still have two of them in a drawer somewhere, naked and handless. It must have been a terrible war.

Every night, when he finished his shift at SeaPak, my dad stopped by the canteen and bought me peanut butter crackers and a carton of chocolate milk. Mama told him to stop, but he couldn't help himself. He wanted to show how much he loved his boy. When I eat those two things now, in my mouth they turn into one—the milk softening the crackers, the crackers flavoring the milk—and in my mind that taste conjures a boy in short pants, playing in the dirt, waiting for Daddy to come home.

My folks often worked staggered shifts. Mama would wake me up at dawn on summer mornings to take me to my cousins' house on her way to work. I'd lie on a pallet in their living room, the country music station on low, Charlie Rich singing about what goes on behind closed doors. Daddy would pick me up in work clothes stained with grease. Mama would come home smelling like shrimp.

My parents never got an education because their families needed them in the fields. Daddy stopped school in sixth grade, and Mama quit after one day of the fourth. But they both loved to read. My dad alternated between his two sacred texts: the Bible and the Bass Pro Shops catalog. My mom, to this day, reads two or three romance novels a week. All that reading rubbed off on me. Somehow I could read and write a little by the time I was two and a half, and I could name every car on the road by sight. The woman who ran the kindergarten next door found out about this and called the *Brunswick News*, the local paper. They came and did a story on me. My mom, of course, still has the clipping. "Tommy's favorite pastimes are reading and writing," the story says. "He spends a lot of time at his blackboard." Today it's a keyboard, not a blackboard, but my life is basically the same.

When I started school, I was ahead of most of the others in

class but way behind on the playground. Donald Evans, the fastest kid in first grade, invented a sport that gave him endless entertainment: He'd slap me on the back of the head and dash out of reach, knowing I could never catch him. I couldn't pull myself up on the monkey bars or clamber up into the live oaks in the schoolyard. (There was a time when schools let kids climb trees. This was before the invention of lawyers.)

The worst days were the ones with relay races. Even now the thought of them makes me sweat with dread. The teachers split us into two long lines. One kid at a time in each line, run to the pine tree and back. As soon as we lined up, kids would shift around to match up with somebody in the other line. I always ended up across from a girl named Pamela. She was as big as me. I'd glance at her, over in the other line, and she looked like I felt—full of fury and scared enough to pee her pants. I never ran harder in my life than during those relay races. I knew I was fat and slow, but I hated being the fattest and the slowest. I wanted to beat Pamela so bad. Sometimes I did, and I am ashamed of how much I enjoyed it. Other times she beat me and ruined my day. Either way, the same thing always happened: When we tagged the tree and turned toward home, the other kids would be laughing at us. Sometimes I wonder where Pamela is, and if she watches the relays at the Olympics, and catches a sudden smell of pine sap, and feels an ache in her gut.

No matter how much I do in life, no matter how far I've made it, it takes only an instant to snap me back to that field of dirt and sandspurs, churning as hard as I can go, still falling behind. All of a sudden I hear that elementary school laughter in my head, and know in my heart, despite all the evidence, that I am back in last place. I have felt that way with teachers and bosses, strangers and lovers. Out of nowhere, sometimes, I start heaving tears. I cry quicker and harder than a man ought to. As big as I am, it takes so little to make me feel small.

Grown-ups never made sense when it came to food. We ran laps in Midget League baseball to get in shape, but if we won a game, we got free snow cones from the concession stand. The go-to flavor was suicide, which was all the flavors mixed together. It tasted brown. When I was nine, and we won the first-half championship, the coach took us all to the Sizzler. I think it was the first time I'd ever been to a steak house. At the end of the season, when we had our team banquet at a fancy place called Bennie's Red Barn, the coach got up to praise us one by one. "And Tommy—well, Tommy's still over there eating," he said, laughing. I looked up from my country-fried steak and noticed that everyone else had put their forks down. Where I came from, somebody talking was no reason to stop chewing.

I don't remember making the connection back then between eating and getting fat. My first side hustle was selling Now & Laters—packs of taffy cut into little squares like Starburst. To South Georgia third graders, they might as well have been crack. I'd buy a pack of ten for a quarter at the little store near our house, then sell the squares for a dime apiece on the playground. I spent some of my profits on comic books but most of it on junk food for myself—Tom's potato chips and Dreamsicles and tiny wax Coke bottles with little shots of fruit drink inside. Scientific studies have shown that there's almost no limit to the amount of sweetness a child likes. I floored the sugar pedal. Sometimes I wonder if little grains of Pixy Stix are still wedged in my cells, waiting to get sweated out.

During the week, my folks didn't have time to cook much. We ate what poor folks ate in the South. Hamburger Helper. Chicken potpies, ten for a dollar at Pantry Pride. Jell-O with fruit cocktail suspended inside and Cool Whip on top. Light bread smeared with Bama peanut butter and jelly, swirled together in one jar so you didn't have to buy two.

What we ate more than anything was fish and seafood. My folks could get frozen shrimp from SeaPak for a dollar a pound. In the eighties, when trendy restaurants started selling shrimp and grits for twenty bucks a plate, it sounded to me like a prank on the Yankees. Shrimp and grits was what we ate if there was nothing else left in the house.

Sometimes we'd catch whiting off the St. Simons pier, or spot-tail bass—what they call redfish or red drum in other places—from the jetties on the beach. But we spent a lot more time in fresh water, mostly in the Altamaha River, which cuts a diagonal slash through southeast Georgia. My dad grew up on the river. He knew every bend in the channel and every overflow pond back in the woods. He had scraped up the money to buy a used bass boat, the fiberglass colored pale green like the hallway of an elementary school. We spent many a Saturday casting balsa-wood plugs and Dedly Dudly spinnerbaits among the cypress knees, looking for largemouth. One morning I pulled in a nine-pound bass on a black plastic worm. We didn't mount it on the wall—we took it home, sliced it into strips, and fried them up like chicken tenders.

But bass were mostly for sport. When we needed to eat, we went for catfish. Five or six kinds lived in the river, and they all tasted different. Mud cats were the worst, then yellow cats, then blues. We wanted channel cats—they lived in moving water, instead of dead spots or eddies, so they weren't as fatty. We'd tie our boat to a willow tree, bait the hooks with worms we dug that morning, and drop a line over the side until the sinker thumped the bottom. If we picked the right spot, within seconds we'd feel the stuttering pull of a channel cat. The younger, smaller ones tasted best. On good days we'd take home a coolerful.

Saturday night at our house, pretty much any weekend between 1970 and 1982: I'm out back with Daddy, skinning catfish and trying to keep from getting finned. (Catfish have fins as sharp as ice picks.) Mama is inside with the skillet, heating drippings from a can on the back of the stove, or maybe a scoop of Crisco. She dredges each fish in cornmeal, then places it in the skillet. If you asked me to narrow my whole childhood into one sensory wash, this is it: the hot bubbles outlining the fresh fish, the grease popping like angry rain, the smell of old river bottom and bacon once removed.

I ate thousands of those fish and have yet to taste anything better. Catfish, french fries, coleslaw, hush puppies, sweet tea. If I ever end up on the Green Mile, that's my last meal.

Everybody in my family was an artist when it came to Southern food. The women cooked the most, but the men could swing a meal now and then—Daddy's specialty was chicken and dumplings, with the dumplings made from crumbled-up soda crackers. The show of the year was the family reunion at Uncle Ted and Aunt Estelle's house in Nahunta, Georgia, which is known (if it is known) for once hosting the World Armadillo Olympics. Uncle Ted worked in the pulp mills and played country blues on his guitar. Aunt Estelle, my dad's sister, was rough as a cob. From the time I was about ten, every time we showed up, she'd take one look at me and holler: "You ain't lost no weight!" And then she would call us to the kitchen, where we would add our dishes to heaven's buffet.

Most of the time, the center of the table was a platter of fried chicken piled so high it would topple if you pulled out the wrong leg. There'd be pork chops, turkey and dressing, beef stew, maybe venison if it was hunting season. Then the white food group: mashed potatoes, potato salad, deviled eggs, rice with brown gravy. Biscuits and cornbread shining with butter. And then the vegetables: crowder peas and Kentucky Wonder pole beans, crookneck squash and fried okra, turnip greens in salty potlikker, sliced tomatoes picked five minutes ago. This paragraph is as close as I will ever come to writing porn.

There was no way to get all the goodness on one plate. Anywhere my family gathered, a normal meal was two helpings. Three if you hadn't tried the meat loaf. If you stopped after one, somebody would ask if you were sick.

The desserts were off to the side on a counter. Somebody would have set out dessert plates, but most of us used our regular plates for the extra room, not caring if the carrot cake soaked up chicken grease. We'd have pecan pie, banana pudding, peach cobbler, pound cake as dense and rich as peat moss. One year in the early seventies, one of our cousins, who had moved to Minnesota, brought home her new husband. He was Japanese. I'm pretty sure nobody at that reunion had ever met a Japanese person before that moment, unless it was in the war. He showed up with a cooler of ice cream. We loved him immediately.

After supper was the time of groaning and unbuckled belts: "Time to sit around and sulk," Uncle Ted would say. The women would clean up and gather around the kitchen table. The men would go outside and lean on the bed of somebody's truck, smoking cigarettes or pinching off chaws of Days Work tobacco. As a kid I had a ticket to both worlds, the women and the men, and I'd hang around the fringes, listening to the stories. Sometimes the hero of the outside version was the villain of the inside version. Either way the stories always had pace, suspense, humor, and a lesson at the end. I'm the only one out of my family who makes a living telling stories, but in many ways I'm the worst storyteller in my family. I've spent my life trying to rework my family's magic tricks, to take that sound and that feeling and turn it into words on a page. My kin, without knowing it, created a writer.

Without intending to, they also created a fat boy.

By the time I came around, the people in my family were off the farm, but most of them still worked with their hands and their backs. I was different. I never had to pick cotton or sweat out a shift at the mill. I ran around outside and played ball, but what I really loved was reading books. My soft life had no chance against a Southern supper table. A few people in my family were starting to grow potbellies, but most still had the jobs and the metabolism to burn off big suppers. I didn't, but the food was so good I couldn't stay away. I'd sneak back into the kitchen for an extra chicken leg or a hunk of pie I'd eat out of my bare hand.

The grown-ups would chase me off, but they weren't serious about it. They were proud of what they grew and caught and cooked. None of us had money. But we were wealthy at the table. I ate better than anyone I knew. I also ate more.

My dad's full name was Leonard Milton Tomlinson, but people always called him Tommy, and he figured that's what everybody would call me. So my folks made it official—it's Tommy on my birth certificate, not Thomas or Tom. From then on, I was Little Tommy and he was Big Tommy. It didn't take me long to turn that into a joke. By the time I was twelve, I was bigger than him.

Right around then, in 1976, we moved from St. Simons to the mainland. My mom got hurt on the job at SeaPak—a metal rack fell on her and crushed nerves in her neck and shoulder. My dad had started to get work building houses. They both wanted a calmer life and a place for a garden. So they bought a cinder-block house right on Highway 341 in Sterling, ten miles north of Brunswick. When we moved there, Sterling had a single flashing light. Forty years later, there's a full red light. Progress.

That fall my mom took me to Jane Macon Middle School to sign up for seventh grade. The principal herself enrolled me. The first day of class, my English teacher started talking about how exciting it must be to be starting *eighth* grade. I went up after class and told her there must be a mistake. It turned out I was so big that the principal assumed I was an eighth grader. When they checked my test scores, they let me stay in eighth-grade English. Our teacher, Lillian Williams, told us dirty jokes on the sly and gave me a stack of her daughter's old Beatles singles. She also picked me to play the lead in the production of *You're a Good Man, Charlie Brown*. I sang a solo and made out with two girls in the cast backstage. God bless you, Mrs. Williams.

Our new house had an acre of rich black dirt—the people before us had kept horses. My folks knew all about gardens from their years in the fields. Soon we were swamped with vegetables. Mama canned peas and froze squash and made scuppernong jelly from our grapevine. We ate healthy more days than not. But by then I had a taste for sugar and fat. When we didn't eat it at home, I found other ways.

My freshman year in high school, I started working two jobs. One was at the Jack's Minit Market down at the traffic light. My main task was to load the racks in the long walk-up cooler that ran across the back of the store. I worked in the freezing-cold room behind the racks, wearing a jacket in the middle of summer, just as my folks had done at the seafood plant. Inventory control at Jack's was not exactly precise, and I was out of sight in the cooler, so I'd pop open a cold drink as soon as I clocked in. I tried every potion Coke and Pepsi made, plus Nehis and RC Colas and Gatorade. Some of the first beers I ever drank were in that little room behind the racks. I came out just before the store closed at eleven. Right after we locked up, the nice old woman who worked the counter would go in the office to put the money in the safe. I took those moments to shoplift candy—mainly Chunky bars, which were easy to stuff in my jacket pockets. In bed, I'd gorge on stolen chocolate.

My other job was at the Sunset drive-in theater. I got that job through James Holt, one of the debate teachers at Brunswick High—his mom ran the theater. We specialized in first-run movies on their second run, grindcore horror films, and X-rated flicks with the X taken out. Not many customers at the Sunset cared what was on the screen. The front rows were crawling with kids in station wagons, and the back rows were full of weed smoke and muffled moans. It was a dream job for me: a small but steady paycheck, all the movie passes I wanted, and bushels of free food. I had a cup of Coke I refilled half a dozen times every night, and a bag I kept filled with warm popcorn. (After seeing popcorn "butter" in its unmelted state—it looked like a block of yellow birdshit—I ate my popcorn dry, and have ever since.) We also sold burgers and hot dogs and little pepperoni pizzas. Some nights, when I ran the projector and was the last one around, I'd make myself one of everything. On top of that, Mrs. Holt—who was born in Korea—would often bring in a big bowl of fried rice for the staff. Some nights I'd eat supper at home, then go to the Sunset and have fried rice and popcorn and hot dogs and pizza. I outgrew the company-issued white dress shirts. Mama had to buy me new ones and sew on the Georgia Theater Company patches.

Brunswick had just one big-and-tall store, a place called P.S. Men's Wear. By the time I was in middle school, that's where I had to get my clothes. It was the quietest place I ever shopped—nothing but fat guys and their wives or mamas, everybody's heads dipped in shame. The dressing rooms there were the first time, but far from the last time, that I cried over clothes. Nothing ever fits right when you're fat, and nothing that does fit is ever in style. If it was close, we bought it anyway. There was nowhere else to go.

I was always hell on clothes. My thighs rubbed together and wore through my corduroys, making me chafe in ways no amount of talcum powder would soothe. If I sat down wrong, or bent over funny, I'd rip a hole in the crotch of my jeans. My legs were too big to keep pressed together—I was manspreading before manspreading was a thing—so everybody could see where Mama had patched the holes with scraps of denim or old bandannas. It was Dolly Parton's coat of many colors down there. It's bad enough any time somebody laughs at your crotch. Worse when you're fifteen.

None of this slowed down my eating. At the high school they had a regular lunch line, where they offered the hot meal of the day. But they also had a sandwich line. You picked up a paper bag with the side items—potato salad, an apple, whatever—and then chose a sandwich to put in the bag. Nobody staffed the sandwich line except the woman taking money at the end. It didn't take me long to figure out I could grab a burger AND a barbecue sandwich AND a ham and cheese and stuff them all in the bag, and no one would check. Three lunches in one! Clearly I was a genius.

My lunches were supposed to be free. Our family income was low enough that I qualified for free lunches the whole time I was in school. When I was in elementary school, they didn't think to disguise that from the other kids. At the beginning of every week the teacher would call a few names, and we'd trudge to her desk in our off-brand shoes to get our little blue punch cards. They marked us as sure as scarlet letters. Once it sank in that I was poor, and everybody knew it, I despised those blue cards. By the time I got to middle school, I wouldn't take them anymore. Mama would count out a dollar or two every day so I could buy lunch. I'm sure it hurt our family. Those dollars added up. I didn't care. I was ashamed of enough already.

Later, after my dad got sick and had to quit work, we stood in line for government cheese. It came in long blocks like Velveeta, except in brown institutional boxes. I hated what that cheese said about us. But it was damn good cheese. I carved it off the block in chunks the size of my hand.

Animal House came out my freshman year at Brunswick High. All my friends loved it, and the scene we loved the most was the food fight. Back then my best friend was another freshman named Nick Arbia, who knew where to get pot and was rumored to have had sex. I had never been close to either. Nick and I thought it would be hilarious to have a food fight at our school. Neither one of us was serious about it, but we talked it up a little and the idea got away from us. By the time the day we had picked came around, a Friday in the spring, the whole school knew about it. We sat down in the cafeteria that day and the whole place got quiet. Everybody waited for us to start something. I wasn't about to start anything. I was too scared. It was like that for a minute or two. Then, from out in the courtyard, somebody threw a sandwich that splatted against the window. That was all it took. All of a sudden pizza slices and fruit cups flew everywhere. I never threw a thing, just hid under a table until it was over. Afterward, I walked back toward class, scared and giddy. Other kids were high-fiving me. I was a fat freshman with acne and crooked teeth, but for a minute I was a hero.

I had just made it through the breezeway and into the next building when someone spun me around. I never saw the punch coming—it caught me flush in the left eye. It staggered me but I didn't go down and I went after him. Then somebody else hit me from the side and knocked me down. The two of them kicked me in the face until a couple of teachers broke it up. It turned out the first guy was the star running back on the football team, and the other was a starter in basketball. Somebody had hit the football player with an apple in the food fight. He and his buddy took it out on me. It's the only real fight I've ever been in. I expect to retire with a lifetime record of 0-1.

It happened to be Fifties Day at school, and I had worn a white T-shirt like the Fonz. Never a good fashion choice, but especially not that day. The front was soaked in blood from my busted nose. They hauled all three of us to the principal's office. We all got suspended—me for the food fight, them for the real one. The principal, a big sports fan, was worried most about the football player. He had hurt his knuckles punching me.

My mom came and picked me up. She drove me home in fury and tears. I couldn't begin to explain what had happened—not right then, anyway. We got home and she cleaned me up and I realized: With all that food flying around my head, I never did get any lunch.

I was hungry.

That was the only really bad thing that happened to me in high school. There were so many good things. I found my tribes—the debate team, the Model UN, the kids who partied but still studied. Three great teachers—James Holt, Brenda Hunt, and Wayne Ervin—praised my work and pushed me to do better. I devoured books despite having to trudge through Thomas Hardy and Theodore Dreiser and those other novelists devised by English teachers in order to make kids hate reading. In my little group I even, to my surprise, found girls who were attracted to me. I spent more Friday nights than I expected out at the edge of the marsh, on a dark cul-de-sac in an unbuilt development called River Ridge, steaming up the windows of my '71 Buick LeSabre. It was a big car. There was plenty of room in the backseat.

(Sex was always such a surprise. I saw myself in the mirror. I knew what I looked like. Even in the moment, in the sweat and the sighs, part of me would think: *You've seen me up close, right? Are you sure about this?*)

Things were good at home, too. I was lucky beyond words to grow up in a stable house with two parents who loved me. I made almost all A's and went to Glyndale Baptist with my folks every Sunday morning. The worst trouble I ever got into was the first night I got drunk, which also happened to be the first night I puked after getting drunk. It was supposed to be an overnight party, but it broke up early and a friend took me home. I opened the door at three in the morning, bumfuzzled and shirtless, to find my mom and dad playing rummy with Uncle Hank and Aunt Hazel. Daddy gave me the silent treatment for a few days after that one. He could have beat me with a cypress limb and it wouldn't have hurt as much.

My dad was wearing down by then from fifty years of smoking and all those years of work. He had a stroke and needed surgery to clear out an artery in his neck. His emphysema tethered him to an oxygen tank, and he couldn't walk to the mailbox without giving out. We needed money, so Mama went back to work as a waitress in a hotel diner that eventually turned into a Denny's. She toted trays with that injured neck and shoulder for eighteen years. The nerves down her back still burn. She would come home exhausted and drop into a chair, handing me her apron so I could empty the pockets and count out her tips. My mama and daddy broke their bodies to make lives for themselves, and to give me a better life than the one they had. It hurt their hearts to see me breaking my body over nothing more than second helpings.

The three of us ate most of our meals in the kitchen at a little table with a Formica top, one of those sets that would be charming and retro now. One night I sat down for supper and the aluminum legs of my chair gave way under me, like a horse kneeling to sleep. None of us knew what to say. I got off the floor, bent the legs back into place, and sat down as light as I could. Then I dove back into my food.

They talked to me over and over about losing weight—Daddy in his gentle way, sliding it sideways into a conversation, Mama head-on and blunt. I responded the way most every teenager does: I didn't listen. I knew what they were saying was true—I felt the hurt when some girl I liked laughed at me, or when I hid in the back of the shower in P.E. class, or when I stayed home on prom night. I couldn't parse out what was normal high school drama and what was special to me because I was fat.

By high school I was plenty old enough to make my own choices. Maybe all that chocolate milk and all those crackers, all that fried chicken and banana pudding, set me on a path. But at some point I decided to walk it on my own. It wasn't—isn't—my parents' fault. I understood exactly what I was doing. I felt like two people—the smart kid with a sweet and lucky life, and the fool trying to eat himself to death.

On graduation night at Brunswick High, I drank a beer in the school parking lot as the principal drove by and scowled. I was eighteen, legal drinking age in Georgia back then, supposedly a man.

A few months before that, my dad sat me down in the living room and told me they had done the best they could but they didn't have enough money to send me to college. I'd never seen him that sad. Maybe I could work for a while, he said, take a class or two at the junior college, save enough to pay my own way. I let him finish and told him something he didn't know: They had these things called Pell Grants that could help families like us pay for tuition and books. Between that and a couple of scholarships

I'd won, that might be enough. Daddy let out a long breath and I hugged him. Pell Grants are named for a senator from Rhode Island named Claiborne Pell who died a few years ago. I've never really had heroes. If I did, my mom and dad would be first. Claiborne Pell would be next.

On a Saturday morning in September 1982, I left Brunswick for Athens to start my freshman year at the University of Georgia. I had a ticket to the football game that afternoon, but no one had told me that game traffic around Athens is like Times Square on New Year's Eve. I didn't get to the city limits until the third quarter. So I listened to the great UGA announcer Larry Munson call the game on the radio as the Dawgs finished off BYU. On the way to the friends' apartment where I was spending the night, I stopped at McDonald's for a burger and the liquor store for a six-pack of Mickey's malt liquor. Mickey's came in grenade-shaped green bottles. It looked like something a college man ought to drink. It tasted terrible. It was the first of many terrible college beers, and that burger was the first of many terrible college meals.

I had nobody to answer to. I had nobody to catch me raiding the fridge at night. I was 270 pounds and about to get a lot bigger.

JANUARY

I start with a hunk of plastic and a plan.

The hunk of plastic is a Fitbit fitness tracker. The one I have is the cheapest version—the Flex, a black band that goes around my left wrist. There's a little capsule inside that acts as a pedometer.

The display is five white dots on a tiny screen. The more steps I take, the more dots light up. If I hit my goal for the day, the dots dance across the screen and the wristband vibrates. The technology is basically Pong. But it does what I need it to do. It holds me accountable.

The Flex connects to a website where I can log in what I eat every day. That's crucial to my plan. I'll talk a lot more about the diet industry later on, but for now just know what I have come to learn through painful experience: The only thing a trendy diet will help you lose is money. I have come to believe there's just one true plan that works in the long term. I call it the Three-Step Diet:

1. Find a way to measure the calories you eat and drink.
2. Find a way to measure the calories you burn.
3. Make sure that every day, number one is smaller than number two.

This doesn't have to cost you a dime. There are loads of free tools, online and at the library, to help you count calories in and calories out. I didn't know, until I got serious about keeping track, that there's a thing called basal metabolic rate: the calories your body burns just to keep your blood flowing and your lungs pumping air. You can find BMR calculators online, and they're all just a guess— a doctor can get you a more precise reading—but in general, the bigger you are, the more it takes to keep the engine running. I burn somewhere between 2,000 and 3,000 calories a day just to stay alive. Right now I'm a Chevy Tahoe. I'd like to be a Prius.

I paid a hundred dollars for the Fitbit because it makes keeping track easy—the pedometer counts my steps and sends the info via Bluetooth to the Fitbit website. The site also has a place to enter other types of exercise—swimming or biking or whatever. Then I just log in what I eat. It has calorie counts for pretty much everything you can think of, including stuff from most restaurant chains. This is where I found out that one of those little bags of tortilla chips they give you at Chipotle is 570 calories. Which means I no longer take the little bag of tortilla chips at Chipotle.

It makes such a difference—at least it does to me—just to write everything down. I've often told people that one reason I became a writer is that I don't really know what I think until I sketch it out on the page. That's what the Three-Step Diet forces me to do when it comes to food and exercise. It's a daily journal of how much I care about leading a better life.

My goal, for now, is to keep my daily intake about 1,000 calories under my outgo. Theoretically, a pound equals about 3,500 calories—although, as I'll talk about later, scientists disagree about this—so 1,000 calories a day equals 7,000 a week, or about two pounds. If I stick to the goal I could lose about two pounds a week, if I do the math right, and if my body conforms to the statistical averages, and if we even really know how many calories are in a pound to begin with. When you're trying to lose weight, most phrases begin with *if*.

Lots of people take their longest walk of the year on New Year's Day, trying to walk off the mistakes of a lifetime, or maybe just the mistakes of last night. Alix and I start the year with a stroll through NoDa, one of our favorite Charlotte neighborhoods. I find a golf ball and a debit card. Somebody had an interesting New Year's Eve. Then we go home and make field peas and collard greens. It's a Southern tradition on New Year's Day—the peas stand for coins, and the greens for folding money. Most people cook the peas with rice and bacon in a dish called hoppin' John. But we're already making cornbread, cooked in one of my mom's old cast-iron skillets, and we're trying to eat better for the New Year. So we skip the bacon and rice. We wish for wealth in love and willpower.

After a couple days in Charlotte, I go back to Georgia to spend a week with my mom. Alix has to work so I go without her. I'm headed straight into the grief over Brenda's death. It hasn't been even two weeks yet. Everything's still raw. Mama's house is full of peace lilies that people sent for the funeral. They're beautiful to look at, until I remember why they're there.

I spend my fifty-first birthday helping Mama get one more day of distance from Christmas Eve. She goes to bed early and I watch *Life Itself,* the documentary on the film critic Roger Ebert. I admired Ebert for lots of reasons. He was a fat guy who thrived on TV through the force of his talent. He wrote about big ideas for a mass audience—something I've always tried to do. He poured out thousands of reviews and books and features and blog posts. He kept working through his terrible battle with cancer and its complications. I've always wanted to be more prolific in life—to write more stories, go more places, have more adventures. At the end, Ebert's whole lower jaw was missing, but he was still churning out words and making the most of his life. Sometimes I think I make the least of mine.

People are still bringing food to Mama's house. There's a pan of baked spaghetti in the fridge, a couple of pies of unknown origin on the counter. I drive down to Brunswick to see my best friend, Virgil Ryals, and his mom. Mrs. Ryals bakes cakes that are restaurant quality. She sends me back with a slab of red velvet and a hunk of pound cake. It's a forty-five-minute drive back to Jesup and they rest on a plate in the passenger seat, whispering their aromas in my nose. I feel like a drug mule moving cocaine up I-95. I could pull over and eat it all and Mama would never know. I make it back without touching the plate. It feels like a huge victory.

But I'm also finishing up a big piece for ESPN, and my nerves always kick in just before a big story comes out. It doesn't matter that I've been doing this for thirty years. I still worry that there's some huge error none of us caught. I worry that nobody will read the story. Most of all I worry that I didn't capture the truth, that it slid out from under me when I looked away. When I get back home, the fear balls up in my gut. On Tuesday afternoon, after Alix goes to work, I go to McDonald's. For the next few days I dive off the wagon.

At the end of the month, I weigh in at our local Y. We don't use the Y nearly as much as we should—I did the math one time and we were paying something like thirty bucks a visit based on our monthly fees. Its main feature for me is the scale in the basement. It goes up to five hundred pounds. You can't buy a normal scale at the store that goes that high—usually they have them just at doctor's offices. This scale is the only one I have access to that fits me.

It has been an up-and-down month—more good than bad, I think, but I don't know for sure. I hate reducing my life to a number. But right now, this number matters.

I step on the scale and watch the digits roll like a slot machine. Anything less than a month ago and I'm a winner.

The numbers stop.

I'm winning. So far.

Weight on December 31, 2014: 460

Weight on January 31, 2015: 455

For the month: -5

For the year: -5

Two

THE COST OF FREE DOMINO'S

My first roommate at UGA, in the Russell Hall dorm, was a junior named Matt. He had regular epic fights with his girlfriend followed by volcanic makeup sex. The legend went that he hadn't changed his bedsheets his entire time in college. You could see the oily outline of his body on the fitted sheet. We called it the Shroud of Matt.

This is only about the fifty-third weirdest story from my four years in Athens, Georgia.

My tribe at UGA formed the first day on campus. I ran into a guy named Jon Bauer—we'd gotten to know each other at a summer academic program the year before. That first day in Athens, Jon was hanging out with some of his friends from his hometown of Albany, Georgia. I was with some of my friends from Brunswick. We added three or four others we met along the way and ended up with a pack of about a dozen. We ate together and drank together and went to movies together, and we often ended the night crammed together in a dorm room, flirting and bullshitting and passing around a cardboard box of popcorn. Sometimes our buddy Zane Vanhook would pull out his guitar and we'd all sing Journey's "Stone in Love."

The whole town was jacked up with energy—intellectual, sexual, musical, and pharmaceutical. The one great thing (the Shroud of) Matt did for me was hand me a record called *Chronic Town*, the newly released first album by a local band called R.E.M. The record sounded dark and murky and confused, which was perfect, because back then I felt dark and murky and confused. We caught R.E.M. before the world knew who they were, when they hung out at the Gyro Wrap or played secret shows under the name Hornets Attack Victor Mature. I've never met them—except for nodding to Pete Buck, the guitar player, while we peed side by side in the men's room at the 40 Watt Club—but they were ours, like cousins who went off and got famous.

My friends and I ate most of our meals at Bolton Hall, known to students as Revoltin' Bolton. These days a lot of universities have dining halls that are like food courts at an upscale mall. Bolton was more like a Soviet cafeteria. We mocked the battered slabs of cod and iffy institutional burgers. Our buddy Todd Waters declared that the *au jus* in roast beef au jus was French for "without taste." But the food was all-you-can-eat and we were all young and hungry. We topped off the meals with the one sure bet in the dining hall—fresh ice cream from the on-campus dairy.

But that wasn't enough for me.

Across the street from our dorm was the Classic Subshop, named after Athens, the Classic City. The subs were the opposite of classic—just a half-step above roast beef without taste—but the beer was cheap and the owner was a sweet guy who always said "Thank you now" as he handed over my microwaved ham and cheese. I went over there three or four times a week. This was before ATM cards—God, I'm old—so if I was broke, I'd cash a check at the gas station next door. The smallest check they'd let you cash was $10.50—they kept the fifty cents as a fee. My quarterly bank statement would have three or four checks for books and tuition, and twenty checks for $10.50. Pretty soon, $10.50 at a time, I drained the money I'd saved that summer and the little bit left over from my Pell Grant. I'd call home on Saturdays, catching up on news from home and making sure I told Mama and Daddy I loved them before I eased into the plea for cash. A few days later, I'd get an envelope with a stack of Mama's tip money. I walked around with a billfold full of one-dollar bills, like some dude getting ready to hit the strip clubs. I converted those bills into a couple thousand extra calories every day.

A lot of that was alcohol. These days I don't drink much—a glass of good bourbon with a little ice, or a cold beer after cutting the grass. But Athens is a twenty-four-hour rolling party if that's what you want, and back then that's what I wanted. We chugged Natural Light from red Solo cups at frat parties, slammed Beam-and-Cokes before football games, downed trays of screwdrivers on Drink 'n' Drown night at a bar called the Mad Hatter. On weekends we'd buy a six or twelve of decent beer—Bud or Miller—and back that up with Drewrys, which went for five bucks a case and had a unique flavor profile: gym socks soaked in untreated sewage. We'd get buzzed on the good stuff and then switch to Drewrys when our tongues went numb. This was also the time Coors went on sale east of the Mississippi. It seems weird now, because nobody actually drinks Coors except in TV commercials, but at the time it was a big deal. (The whole plot of *Smokey and the Bandit*, that cinema classic from 1977, revolves around Burt Reynolds escorting a truckload of bootleg Coors from Texas to Georgia in his black Trans Am.) When Coors arrived in Athens, you couldn't buy cans or bottles—just kegs. A couple of smart liquor stores started selling it by the gallon. I'd see guys walking back to the dorms with Coors in milk jugs. This might have been the invention of the growler.

Drinking felt like bonding. It also gave me courage. If I had enough to drink, I might be brave enough to slip my hand onto a girl's bare thigh at a party. If she had enough to drink, she might let me leave it there. After two or three Long Island iced teas, I felt charming and suave. That was a big improvement over most of the time, when I felt enormous and unattractive.

Of course, once the morning came, all that booze made me even more enormous and unattractive.

Besides drinking, my other hobby was basketball. Our group played for hours on the Russell Hall outdoor slab most every afternoon and night. (My dear friend David Duclos is hoping I don't mention the time Joe Ward, a UGA star slumming on our court after getting kicked out of practice, spiked one of David's jumpers all the way across Baxter Street into the Krystal parking lot. Sorry, bud.) Sometimes we'd play until midnight or later, pissing off the students in the dorm who were actually studying. One night a guy shot bottle rockets at us from his window. But we had another reason to stay up. Jon Bauer worked delivering Domino's, and at the end of the night they'd split up the leftover pizzas—ones where they had gotten the order wrong, or somebody didn't pay. He'd come back at one in the morning with two or three pizzas in hand. We never had pizza delivered to the house when I was growing up. The idea of somebody bringing you pizza felt like a gift just by itself. But *free* pizza, in the middle of the night? God almighty. We'd sprawl out in a dorm room, sweaty and exhausted, downing greasy slices while respectable students slept. It was better than found money on the street.

Free pizza, cheap beer, microwave subs, unlimited ice cream. That was my diet my first year in college. All the basketball in the world wouldn't have burned off those calories. The normal freshman fifteen became my freshman forty.

Over the next couple of years I settled into a life of half-assery. I half-assed my studies, half-assed the few dates I managed to score, half-assed figuring out my future. I blew off classes, coasting on good memory and a way with essay questions. My A's drifted into B's and C's, then into an eddy of incompletes. I declared my major as prelaw, because I had to put down something, but the only thing I knew about my career was that I absolutely did not want to be a lawyer. Lawyers wore suits.

As a freshman I had written a couple pieces for the *Red & Black*, UGA's student newspaper. One of the stories was about an expensive rug the university bought for one of the administration buildings. When somebody at the university complained about the story, I got spooked and quit. But the rush of writing a story, then seeing it published, buzzed in my blood. My mom and dad had subscribed to the *Brunswick News* as far back as I could remember. When I was a kid, I'd listen for the thump of the paper landing in our yard every afternoon. I'd run out and grab it and peel off the green rubber band so we could split up the sections. I was always curious about how the world worked—how the cops figured out who broke into somebody's house, how the bridge over the river got built, why the Atlanta Braves kept losing every year. All those years of reading, and all those family stories, made me better at writing than anything else. I was built to be a journalist—I just hadn't figured it out. In my junior year, I went back to the *Red & Black*. I wrote a story, then another, and that's all it took. It felt like dancing with a lover. So long, prelaw.

College newspapers always have people coming and going, so if you stick around you get promoted fast. Within a few weeks I became a senior writer. It was a paying gig—three hours a week at minimum wage, even though I was working thirty. We got paid every other week. My first newspaper paycheck, sometime in the fall of 1984, was for eleven bucks and change. I've written for a living ever since.

As my workload at the paper rose, my GPA sank in direct proportion. Every quarter I booked my classes to be done by noon. After class I'd have a burger and beer for lunch at a bar called the Odyssey, then head over to Jackson Street to the newspaper office. There's an old line journalists use: *We don't put out the newspaper, it escapes.* Every day it felt like the *Red & Black* barely got out the door.

Until my senior year, we worked on typewriters. One spot in the middle of the newsroom floor was so rotten that we covered it with a traffic cone so nobody would fall into the Kinko's below. It was an independent paper, not controlled by the university, although we did have a faculty adviser nobody listened to. One day he stomped up the stairs screaming, "WHO THE FUCK THOUGHT IT WAS OKAY TO PUT *FUCK* IN THE PAPER?"

I banged out hundreds of stories and columns, most of them terrible, because most of us are terrible at anything before we get good. But once I started doing journalism I never wanted to do any other kind of work. I still can't believe it's a real job you can get paid for. We get to talk to people and find stuff out and tell the world about it. That's the job at its core. *Guess what I heard today? Holy shit, you're not gonna believe it.*

As much as I loved the paper, it made my bad habits worse. We worked every night until eight or nine and had late, boozy suppers, usually chili and margaritas from Gus Garcia's across the street. Most of my clothes didn't fit anymore. For a while, I had outgrown just about everything but a white sweatshirt and a dishwater-gray bathing suit that I declared to be shorts. I wore that ensemble three or four times a week for months. It's stunning that I didn't hook up with more hot college girls.

I'd moved off-campus with a few buddies by then, first to a couple of apartments, then to an old house on Oconee Hill that was missing its back stairs—it was a ten-foot drop straight down from the back door. Somehow nobody ended up splatted on the ground at one of our parties. On Saturdays we'd head out on Atlanta Highway to Sonny's, a Southern barbecue chain. They had an all-you-can-eat deal on weekends and we'd leave the place in ruins. Well, Sonny's might not have been in ruins. Our stomachs definitely were. My favorite time of the week was Sunday during NFL season. The games started at 1:00, and I'd wake up about 12:55, take a leak, grab cold pizza and leftover beer from the fridge, and watch football until I fell asleep on the couch. Other days I'd have happy-hour bar food, take-out subs, or spaghetti at home washed down with knockoff Coke from Kroger. It was twenty-five cents for a two-liter bottle, and overpriced.

David and Zane had generous parents who would come to Athens sometimes and take us all out to eat. The big place to go in Athens back then was Charlie Williams Pinecrest Lodge, out in the woods a couple miles from town. Charlie Williams served family-style, and in my memory, everything was fried—fried chicken, fried fish, fried pork chops, fried potatoes, fried okra, fried coleslaw (I might be wrong about the slaw). We devoured it all and staggered out into the Georgia night, high on grease and sweet tea.

I thought about food more than classwork, more than the newspaper, more than soft lips in low light. It showed. By the spring of 1986, the end of my senior year, I was on the wrong side of three hundred pounds. That's an educated guess. I wouldn't go to the doctor and I didn't go to the gym. I never wanted to be anywhere near a scale.

My first apartment out of college was a one-room upstairs unit behind a dry cleaner's in Augusta, Georgia. A king-sized bed took up just about the whole room. The landlord had squeezed in a couple of dressers and a mini-fridge. There was no way to cook—not even a microwave. The guy in the apartment next to mine was a boxer, or wanted to be—he hung a heavy bag on his balcony and banged on it for hours. The rest of the time, he and his girlfriend banged on the bed that backed up to my wall. That was my entertainment—pounding of one kind or another—as I watched baseball alone and ate takeout fried chicken from a place called WifeSaver.

It was the summer of 1986 and I was working for the *Augusta Chronicle* and *Herald*, the first and only place that had offered me a job out of UGA. They were two newspapers, the *Chronicle* in the morning and the *Herald* in the afternoon. You wrote the story for one paper then moved the words around a little bit for the other. The editor in chief had taught at Washington and Lee, so we had a bunch of reporters from Washington and Lee. He also liked beautiful redheads, so we had more than our share of beautiful redheads.

My first beat was night cops reporter, three to midnight, chasing every car wreck and armed robbery in a county of almost two hundred thousand people. In Athens I had written about university politics and frat parties. In Augusta I saw a motorcycle cop take off his shoes, dive into a canal, and pull a drowning boy from the bottom. I called mothers of teenagers who'd just been murdered, letting them talk through their tears and asking to borrow a photo. One day I drove way out to the east side of town to cover a wreck. I got there and saw that a woman had run her car into the back of a logging truck. One of the logs went through her windshield. The EMTs cut a hole in the top of the car and tried to lift her out, but they couldn't get a good hold and her shirt came up over her head. She hung there for a second, lifeless and topless, until they could get her out and make her decent.

Every other day I thought I might get fired. I accidentally put a police officer's home address in a story. One night I rewrote a story from scratch instead of going into the version the editor had already worked on. It caused her an extra half hour of work on a brutal deadline. She sent a letter to the city editor that night saying I didn't have what it took for the job. But they kept me around and finally, slowly, I got better. The editors promoted me to the politics beat and let me write features on the side. I did one piece about teenagers who took over a shopping center parking lot on Friday nights, cruising a big loop in their cars. A reader wrote in to say she knew the story wouldn't be any good just by looking at my byline: Tommy was a "childish euphemism" (instead of Thomas or Tom, I guess). For the next couple of months, my nickname around the newsroom was Childish Euphemism.

Back then, at least there, it was still considered OK for newspaper people to have a drink or two at lunch. Some days we'd walk down the street to a place called the Sports Center for beer in frosted fishbowl glasses, plus burgers from the griddle. Wednesday nights we'd go to the Red Lion for $1.50 pitchers. Fridays we'd drink gin-and-tonics at a hotel bar that was so dark we called it the Batcave. When I worked night cops, some nights I'd wait around for the guys in the pressroom to finish up and we'd cross the Savannah River to North Augusta, South Carolina, where bars could stay open all night. Augusta is a big hospital town, and once or twice I saw nurses stop by for a quick beer at sunrise on their way into work. I decided not to get sick in Augusta.

One huge perk of working for the Augusta paper is getting to cover the Masters—the most famous tournament in golf and one of the biggest sporting events in the world. Augusta National Golf Club lets commoners visit the course that one week a year, just to watch, but otherwise the place is vacuum-sealed to keep away everybody but the (rich and powerful, mostly white and male) members and their guests. After the Masters is over the club hosts a media day, when newspeople who cover the tournament get a chance to play the course. If you're not into sports, understand this: a round at Augusta National is the golden ticket of golf. Fans consider the course almost a literal cathedral. If you are one of those fans, take a deep breath before you read the rest of this sentence: I played Augusta National wearing Converse high-tops, swinging mismatched clubs I bought at a pawnshop.

I know. I'm sorry.

I was a fairly regular golfer back then, playing with my buddies Andy Marlatt, Kevin Procter, and Robert Naddra at a public course correctly nicknamed the Cabbage Patch. The four of us played Media Day together. Maybe I shouldn't tell this, because I'm not sure if the statute of limitations ever runs out at Augusta National, but at one point Kevin tried to brake his golf cart on the rain-slicked tenth fairway and accidentally threw the cart into a power slide. We thought we might be shot on sight. The course was dumbed down for hackers like us, but I still shot 118—a tidy 46-over. However! On the sixteenth hole—a gorgeous par-three across a pond—I swung my pawnshop three-iron and landed the ball ten feet from the flagstick. I missed the putt, of course, but tapped in for par. It is, and always will be, the athletic highlight of my life. I might have mentioned this to several thousand people since that day.

Those few years in my mid-twenties should've been my physical peak. But I was eating those Sports Center burgers and that Wife-Saver chicken, and staying out late for drinks every night. I might have had a fleeting thought now and then about cutting back, but the moment I got that first chemical jolt of pleasure, the rational part of my brain switched off. One day I was visiting Andy, my golf buddy, and told him I was trying to get in shape. "Maybe you could start by not eating all our candy," he said. I looked down and saw I'd eaten every Hershey's kiss and Reese's cup from the bowl on the end table between us. It was pure reflex. In the back of my mind, as we talked, I knew I was eating candy. I had no idea I was eating *all* the candy.

After three years in Augusta I thought it was time to work for a bigger and better paper. North Carolina had some of the best in the country. I lined up interviews in Greensboro and Charlotte. I got to the Greensboro paper early on a Monday morning, only to find out that they had been trying to reach me—this was before cell phones—to let me know they didn't want to interview me after all. The secretary took pity on me and let me fill out a generic application. While I was doing that, the editor walked in and did a double take when he saw me. Clearly I wasn't supposed to be there. He gave me five minutes that were wasted on both of us.

The next day at the *Charlotte Observer* changed my life. The *Observer* is still a fine paper, but in 1989 it was a powerhouse—it had just won a Pulitzer for exposing Jim and Tammy Faye Bakker's scams at the PTL Club. The paper's reach covered both Carolinas. You could buy a copy from the Smoky Mountains to Hilton Head. After the disaster in Greensboro I didn't think I had a chance. But they kept running me through interviews with what seemed like every editor in the building. At some point, a reporter told me that if the editors really wanted me, they'd ask me to stick around for another set of interviews the next day. They asked me to stick around. I was too wired to stay in my hotel room that night. I scanned the paper to figure out what was going on in town, and saw that Buckwheat Zydeco was playing at a blues club called the Double Door. I went over there, walked in the back, and saw Bill O'Connor, one of the editors I had met with that day. He was drinking beer and playing foosball. In that moment, I knew I was home.

The *Observer* put me in a one-person office in Lancaster, South Carolina, forty miles south of Charlotte. The paper had a bureau up the road in Rock Hill, and my office was a bureau of *that* bureau—a subatomic particle of journalism. That September, three months after I took the job, Hurricane Hugo wrecked the South Carolina coast and churned right up Interstate 26, far deeper inland than anyone expected. At some point it became clear that Hugo would hit the Charlotte area at nearly full strength. I dozed off watching the weather on TV. The hurricane woke me up at three in the morning, screaming through the eaves. I lived in an old duplex and the front door wasn't square in the frame. The wind flung it open and a bucket of rain flew in through the screen. This happened three times, until I grabbed my old Royal typewriter—a gift from my mom and dad—and jammed it against the base of the door. There was a pecan tree outside my bedroom window, and every new blast of wind bent it over the roof of the house, like a hammer clawing a nail from a two-by-four. The power had gone out and all I could see was the silhouette of the tree in the blur of the rain. I could hear it creak and crack. I wondered if this would be how I died. But the tree held, and the front door held, and around sunrise the wind trailed off. I walked outside and started filling my notebook.

I made some lifelong friends at the paper right away. While I was writing about Lancaster school board meetings, my buddy Joe Posnanski was writing about high school volleyball games for the Rock Hill office. Now he's one of the best and most popular sportswriters in the country, author of the best-selling biography of Joe Paterno. We've done OK for two boys from the bureaus. But outside of work, I spent my time in Lancaster trying not to be lonely, and failing. I struck out the few times I tried to socialize in town. I lived alone and worked alone and it brought out all my worst habits. My office was littered with fast-food bags—I didn't even have the gumption to throw them in the trash can. One of the paper's advertising reps stopped by the office one day to use the phone and was so disgusted she reported me to my boss. I worked a lot of late nights, and sometimes the only place open on the way home was Hardee's. One night I ordered half a dozen cinnamon biscuits at the drive-through. The cashier raised her eyebrows when I came around to pay. I told her they were for my dog. She knew I was full of shit. She laughed in my face and pushed the biscuits through the window.

That Christmas, it snowed in Brunswick. We got a trace of snow every four or five years down there—just enough to get a flake on your tongue—but this time it snowed for real, four inches. I made angels in the yard and threw snowballs at Mama on the porch. Daddy watched from the window. The emphysema had just about stolen his breath. He had worked fifteen-hour days in cotton fields, cut down pine trees in the Georgia swamp, built houses from a pile of lumber and nails. Now our little house was his whole world. He was so glad to see me come home. He told a couple of his favorite old jokes and we watched wrestling on TV. He never could understand how Ric Flair could get away with cheating like he did.

A couple weeks later, after I had gone back to work, he went in the hospital. He had been admitted half a dozen times since I was in middle school, but this time felt different. I came back to see him in the ICU, and he was a fraction of the man I'd just spent Christmas with. He recognized me at first but then he drifted away. He kept reaching into the space between us, grabbing at something in the empty air. He said they were spoons. He asked me if I saw spoons.

On January 8, 1990, four days after my twenty-sixth birthday, Mama was in the ICU with him when he rose up, drew one big breath, then fell back and died. I was in the waiting room, not thirty feet away.

My belly, in a weird way, is a monument to the incredible feat that he and Mama pulled off. They survived the cotton fields and scraped together a better life through hard work and good sense and kindness. They raised a boy who never had to worry about having enough to eat. That has caused its own problems. But I would take these problems every day over the ones they had to face. Just one generation ago, my people rode to town in a wagon and used an outhouse. Now I have a closet full of clothes and a frequent-flier account. It is only fair, in some ways, that I haul this weight around. My mom and dad carried the heavy end of the load long before I got here.

Every so often, my dad shows up in a dream. He never says a word. He doesn't need to. He knows I know.

I spent the next couple years feeling sorry for myself. Looking back, I was doing a lot better than I thought. Some of my stories started landing on the front page of the main *Observer*. I got a promotion to the Rock Hill office to write a column. I ended up with my first girlfriend in years, a woman from the Lancaster paper who had long legs and loved the blues. But I kept expecting to get promoted to the Mothership—the main office in Charlotte—and it didn't happen. Other reporters got called up before me. One of them, Paige Williams, now writes for the *New Yorker*, and another, Carol Leonnig, has gone on to win three Pulitzers with the *Washington Post*. So my bosses were probably right. But I thought my career had stalled out. So I thought about it—not nearly long enough—and then I walked in one day and quit. I left my friends puzzled and my girlfriend hanging. All I could think about was how the paper was holding me back. I threw myself a going-away party and puked up the remnants the next morning. My friend Perry helped me load up the U-Haul. We drove to Atlanta and I moved in with Virgil—my other best friend from home—and his roommate Randy Lockey. A former coworker had a connection with the Cartoon Network. I'd get a job there, freelance on the side, set the city on fire.

It did not go that way. I wrote a couple pieces for magazines, but the only steady job I had the whole time was chasing down high school football scores for the Atlanta paper every Friday night. I rode the last MARTA train home with a group of drag queens. At least I learned a few things about fashion. I spent my little paychecks on chili dogs from the Varsity and fried chicken from Mrs. Winner's. Virgil and I started playing tennis again—we had played each other since high school. He had gotten better and I had gotten slower. One night we decided to play a set. I went up 5-love. But then his big serves started going in, and every time I came to the net he'd drop a lob over my head. I was too slow to run them down. He came all the way back and won. I threw my racket over the fence. I was furious because I kept losing, and not just in tennis.

I had saved some money but it ran out fast. I was still making payments on a used Chrysler LeBaron convertible I'd bought the year before I quit the paper. At one point I got way behind on the payments and started getting calls from a collection agency. I had to drive out to an office park in Cobb County to make a payment. The office was closed off from the public—you rang the bell and they talked to you through a speaker. They had demanded a payment in cash. I was so tapped that I had to use the coins from my change jar. I pushed a wad of bills and some rolls of pennies through the slot in the door. I could hear the agents on the other side of the wall laughing at me.

A couple weeks after that, I called the *Observer* and asked to come back. I would have begged if I'd had to. I was broke, and my mom was having a hard time without my dad. Our old garden back home was overgrown with weeds. I needed to take care of myself, and to take care of her if I needed to. The paper took me back with grace. They had an opening at the Mothership for a feature writer. I was thrilled to take it. I started just after New Year's 1993. By then I must have been 350 pounds.

I moved into a little fourplex a mile or so from the office and started reconnecting with old friends. I promised myself that this time I'd eat right. I started taking long walks around my new neighborhood, grateful for another chance.

Everything felt right. Except for one thing. I had a rasp in my voice that wouldn't go away.

FEBRUARY

We take our dog to the vet and talk about the end. Fred, our yellow Lab mix, is almost fourteen. Arthritis makes his back legs so stiff that he goose-steps down the sidewalk—one of our neighbors calls him Little Soldier. Sometimes he topples over and waits for one of us to pick him up.

On top of all that, he has started turning away from his food and throwing up what he does eat. Dr. Mary Fluke, our amazing vet, loves on him and gives him a cookie and diagnoses a kidney infection. The medicine makes him feel better but doesn't solve his bigger problems. We ask her how to know when it's time to let him go. She says we need to ask five questions:

Does he eat and drink OK?
Can he control his pee and poop?
Can he get around on his own?
Is he engaged with the world?
Does he seem happy?

Getting around is hard, but he's eating better and is OK on everything else. So we give him a wishful five-for-five.

That night, as Alix sleeps beside me and Fred snores on the floor, I turn those five questions on myself.

Do I eat and drink OK?

I'm great at eating and drinking. It's what I do best. I need to figure out how not to be so good at it.

Can I control my pee and poop?

One of the things about being fat is that your belly mashes down on your bladder, so I have the bladder of a chipmunk. Every night I get up two or three times and stumble to the bathroom. I pee before going into a movie and after coming back out. I pee twice at the airport before I get on a plane. Plus, these days, I'm drinking more water to get in shape. I might as well keep a urinal strapped to my crotch.

My other charming bodily function is fairly constant gas. Sometimes I try to hold it in and it rumbles around inside me. Alix has nicknamed it the troll. The troll tends to come out at the most awkward times, like when we're trying to have a romantic dinner. *Excuse me, honey. Keep the candle lit while I go squeeze out a couple of gigantic farts.* My stomach is such an asshole.

Can I get around on my own?

As long as I don't have to run, or go up a lot of steps, or walk a really long way. This is exactly how the average ninety-year-old would answer this question. Shit.

Am I engaged with the world?

My job puts me in interesting places and forces me to talk to strangers. One of my theories about journalism is that it attracts wallflowers, because the job makes us get out on the dance floor. Alix and I visit our families. We go out with friends. But I work from home and a lot of days I don't see or talk to anyone after my wife leaves for the office. Inertia kicks in, and I dick around on the Internet, and here comes four in the afternoon and I still haven't showered. Writers need time alone. It's part of the gig. But sometimes I pull the plug on the outside world and hide. And when I do that, my sustenance is almost always food that's bad for me.

Am I happy?

Yes. Mostly. I hit the wife jackpot, the family jackpot, the friend jackpot, the dog jackpot, and the job jackpot. But my weight locks so many doors. When I run into one of those locked doors, two things happen. First I have a flash of anger—so quick and so deep that Alix will sometimes step back and wonder what the hell just happened. That goes away fast. But then a blue fog lingers—sometimes for five minutes, sometimes for five days. Sometimes it would probably qualify as depression. It involves a lot of staring out of windows. I can't do so many things because I have not done the main thing. And in the blue fog, I hate myself.

Here is the worst thing about addiction: In those lowest moments, what you crave is the very thing that put you in that place to begin with. I am mourning Fred even before he is gone, and it's a cold and bitter February, and I want junk food more than I want anything else in this world. But this time, this February, I take a walk or a shower or drink some water or read a book. And I go back to question one.

Do I eat and drink OK?

A little better now.

Weight on January 31: 455

Weight on February 28: 452

For the month: -3

For the year: -8

Three

THE BEST BAD ROAST
BEEF SANDWICH

We sat in a cold room and the surgeon explained how he would cut my throat.

The larynx is sort of a triangle, he said, sketching a top-down view on a sheet of paper. *We'll have to take off about this much.* He drew a line across a corner of the triangle and most of the way up one side. The line marked off forty percent of my voice box.

We hope you'll be able to talk again, the surgeon said. *But I can't guarantee it.*

This was the beginning of 1993. The paper had hired me back. I had a new job in the Big House as a feature writer, focusing on pop music. I sat next to a theater critic who told great dirty jokes and a movie critic who sang opera in the men's room. My new apartment was five minutes from the office. Everything felt right except for my voice. It sounded like laryngitis but it wouldn't go away.

I went to a regular doctor who gave me a quick exam and shrugged. He sent me to Dr. Donald Kamerer, who I found out later was the best ear, nose, and throat guy in town. He found a polyp in my voice box. They're almost always benign, and he said he could snip it out in outpatient surgery. We made the appointment for a few days later. The surgery went quickly, as he promised. But while I was in the recovery room, Dr. Kamerer took a quick look at the polyp in the lab. He knew I was headed to Georgia to spend time with family while I healed up. As I was being wheeled out the door, he said in sort of an offhand way: *Maybe come back sooner instead of later.*

I tried not to think too hard about what that meant. I didn't want to borrow trouble. But I came back after a long weekend. I made an appointment to meet him at his office down the street from the hospital. And now he was drawing the diagram in that cold examining room and telling me I had squamous cell carcinoma. Throat cancer.

I had just turned twenty-nine.

Most people get throat cancer from smoking. Mama and Daddy were both heavy smokers, but I never smoked and it's rare to get that type of cancer secondhand. Alcoholics get throat cancer. So do people with chronic acid reflux. None of the triggers fit me. When you look at the stats for the causes of any disease, there's a small percentage of people who get it for strange reasons or in unknown ways. They get labeled as Other.

I was Other.

I stumbled out of his office like a zombie and got in my car and cranked the heater up. It didn't cut the cold. I sat there in the parking space and cried.

Dr. Kamerer had said this type of cancer wasn't life-threatening. But that didn't change the fear that was grinding a hole in my gut. They could find more cancer. Something could go wrong and I could die on the table. I'd barely gotten my life started. Part of me was furious at my shitty luck. But part of me thought it must be punishment for getting so fat. Maybe I'd wrecked so much of my life that God was just cutting his losses. *You wanna see a wasted life? I'll show you a wasted life.*

For the thousandth time, I vowed to lose weight and get in shape. This time it came with a coda: *Just let me live.*

I got second and third and fourth opinions on how to get rid of the cancer. In the end, there were two options—surgery or radiation. Radiation would preserve my voice, but there was a smaller chance of getting all the cancer. Surgery would get all the cancer, but there was a chance I would come out the other side with no voice.

I picked surgery. Mute was better than dead. But I wondered what the prospects would be for a reporter who couldn't talk.

During one of my office visits, Dr. Kamerer turned to talk to a nurse and I could see the notes he had taken on my case. Two words jumped out: *morbidly obese.* I'm not sure I had heard that phrase before. It was definitely the first time I had thought about it as a description of me.

In medicine, it's a technical term: somebody who has a body mass index of forty, which usually means at least a hundred pounds more than ideal weight. But there's a literary jolt to the phrase.

Morbid means "dwelling on death." Morbidly obese meant I was so fat that my fat would probably kill me. Unless cancer cut in line.

Because of my morbid obesity, there was some discussion about whether it was safe to do the surgery at all. Anesthesiologists don't like fat patients. It's hard to keep the airway open. Because the surgery was going to be on my throat, they would have to do a tracheotomy. Keeping me breathing and sedated would be complicated. But the morning of the surgery, Dr. Kamerer was calm and positive. They wheeled me in on my back and I looked up at the lights and after a minute or two I went under.

Every hospital recovery room feels the same. Thin curtains between the beds. Nurses in clogs padding around. Some old guy moaning. I woke up with a slash across the left side of my neck, fastened with staples. I breathed through a hole in my throat. Some kind of milky Ensure-looking stuff was being pumped through a tube in my nose. I would end up losing ten pounds in the hospital. The Cancer Diet is surprisingly effective.

They didn't have a hospital gown big enough to fit me. They had to snap two gowns together to make something that ended up looking like Homer Simpson's muumuu. It had to be changed a lot because green gunk drained out of my wound and down the front. I had bought a new red bathrobe to wear over the gown(s). It got funky after a few days so my brother took it to a Laundromat. Ronald doesn't do much laundry. He washed the robe with my whites. So my daily outfit ended up being a gunk-coated double gown, a washed-out bathrobe, and pink underwear. I have yet to see this ensemble at Fashion Week.

I couldn't talk, so I wrote in little spiral notebooks. I wrote notes to the doctor and the nurses and my visiting friends and Mama, who slept beside me almost every night in a chair next to the bed. It's hard to talk in real time on paper. The thoughts come out too fast to write them down. One time I squabbled with Mama over some little thing and chucked my notebook across the room. She let it lie there. That shut me up.

Hospital time, science has proven, moves ten times slower than regular time. Every hour felt like half a day. I couldn't eat, couldn't drink, couldn't shower. I felt like a country ham hanging in a barn, growing mold. A nurse came by and washed me a couple times, which I'm sure was a joy for her. My friends at the paper had bought me a Game Boy and I burned hours playing Tetris. I saw falling blocks on my eyelids when I tried to sleep. My friend Clint Engel came by to watch the Charlotte Hornets' playoff game against the Boston Celtics. It turned out to be the greatest game (so far) in Hornets history—Alonzo Mourning, our six-ten center, hit a long jumper with time running out to win it. His teammates dogpiled on top of him, and the fans at the Charlotte Coliseum went crazy, and Clint jumped and screamed in my room, and all I could do was pump my fist in silence. Somewhere underneath that slash in my neck, my body was deciding if I would ever get to scream and cheer again.

On my seventeenth day in the hospital, they took out the tracheostomy tube. A bunch of doctors and nurses gathered in my room. Dr. Kamerer told me to hold my hand over the hole and try to say something. "One small step for man . . ." would've been nice.

Maybe "Hello, I'm Johnny Cash." But I hadn't thought it through. I was exhausted and scared. Whatever happened next would push my life in one direction or another.

I took the deepest breath I could.

"Hey," I said, and sound came out.

The doctors and nurses cheered. Mama cried.

Greatest word of my life.

After that it was time to undo all the things they had done. A nurse came in and took out all twenty-some staples, one by one, each one pinging into a metal bedpan. The IV came out. The drains with the green gunk came out. At some point they pulled out the feeding tube. I had been sedated when it went in and had no idea how long it was. It felt like a thirty-foot garden hose coming out of my nostril.

Then I got to eat.

Here's what I figure hospitals think about food: If you're in the hospital you might die anyway, so there's no point wasting a good meal on you. Lunch for the patients that day was roast beef sandwiches. Have you ever seen the translucent sheen of gas in a puddle? The roast beef had that sheen. The lettuce on top of it had long since fainted. Even I, in a normal moment, might have taken a pass. This was not a normal moment. I bit off a chunk and chewed. There have been ten thousand better meals in my life. But I've never had a single bite that tasted as good as that little piece of crappy roast beef sandwich.

For a moment it made me forget about the hospital and the scar already itching on my neck and having cancer at twenty-nine and being the Other. A big enough pleasure can push back any pain. I guess I always knew I ate as a salve against the wounds of the world. But it never felt as direct as it did there in the hospital bed. I was alive and could talk and could eat. No pill from God or Pfizer would have made me feel that good.

It took months of voice therapy, blowing on pitch pipes and throat-humming like Billy Bob Thornton in *Sling Blade*, just to build up to the voice I have today—a raspy, thin thing that wears out fast. Some women say it's sexy. To me it sounds like an obscene phone caller in training. At least twice a week for these last twenty-plus years, some stranger has asked if I have a cold, or if I yelled too much at the ball game. Most of the time I just say yes.

In the long run, the limitations of my voice made me better at my job. People had trouble hearing me on the phone, so I got out of the office to see them face-to-face. I couldn't shout at a press conference, so I pulled people over to the side. Most important, because my voice wore out if I talked too much, it made me shut up and listen. I moved in close so people could hear me. It made the conversation more intimate. Even before the surgery, I preferred big stories about little moments. Now I needed those little moments to survive as a writer.

The same lessons crossed over into the rest of my life. I'm useless at a party unless I can get to a quiet place, away from the crowd. The conversation you have on the porch is different than the one you have in a busy kitchen. My voice shapes how I write because it shapes how I live.

I spent the next few years mostly covering concerts. It was a thrill to see great live music and get paid for it. Sometimes it was better to see bad live music and get paid for it. One night I went to see Courtney Love's band Hole. She half-assed the music, did an impromptu audience poll on sexually transmitted diseases, and waved around a stuffed elk head to the point I thought she might impale the bass player. God knows where she got a stuffed elk head to begin with. After I panned the show in the paper, I got a letter from a group of Hole fans that began:

Dear Tommy Tomlinson,

You suck.

And proceeded to list ten reasons why.

A couple years later, in 1996, the paper shuffled some jobs and there was an opening for a local columnist. It was the best job at the paper and something I'd always wanted to try. A bunch of people applied, inside the paper and out. We wrote sample columns and the paper published some of them. Then there were budget problems. Then management indecision. A year and a half went by. I figured that if they were going to pick one of us, they'd have done it already. My friend Joe Posnanski told me about a sportswriting job at the *Kansas City Star*, where he was working at the time. So I flew out there and interviewed. When I got back, the *Observer's* managing editor, Frank Barrows, invited me to breakfast. We met on a Saturday morning at Anderson's, a diner that's now closed but used to be the place where deals got done in Charlotte. I ordered sausage patties and grits. Frank offered me the columnist job. I said yes before he got to the period.

A columnist is the conduit between a paper and its readers. You get to say what you think, praise the praiseworthy, call out corruption and meanness, reveal a little bit of yourself. I was thirty-three and probably one of the youngest local columnists in America. But over time I built a following. People started to notice me on the street. My friends David and Cathy Duclos came to visit one weekend, and when we went out to dinner at LongHorn Steakhouse, we noticed a woman staring at our table. She finally walked over, wobbly from a couple of drinks. She blurted out how much she liked my columns and asked for my autograph. David, who has known me since I was a doofus drunk freshman at UGA, had this astonished expression on his face the whole time: *What the hell is happening?*

There were lots of nice moments like that. I kept expecting somebody to notice me on the street and take a swing at me, but it never happened. Correction: It hasn't happened yet.

When I became a columnist, my picture started running in the paper. In my case it was just a mug shot, but it was enough to show my extra chins. So from day one, every time I had a piece in the paper, I could count on some version of the kids back at elementary school hollering *Fat ass.*

Writing for anyone but yourself requires two skins. One has to be soft and porous, to let the feelings of the story flow through you.

The other has to be solid and flameproof, to shield you from the blowback. Anything you write that matters enough to be loved will also be hated. Most of the letters and emails and phone calls I got as a columnist were kind. Some were criticism I needed—thoughtful disagreement with what I'd said, fair points about things I'd missed, critiques of my style and grammar. One poor retired English teacher beat me with a verbal stick every time I wrote the word *ain't*. But underneath all that was the crawl space where readers went straight for my weakest spot. Some wondered how I dared to judge anybody else when I couldn't keep my own weight under control. Others said they were disgusted to see my face in the morning. One regular would end her letters with a sentence or two about how karma would make things right one day by giving me diabetes or a heart attack. (She was a nurse. I wondered about her patients.) Some days there might be one email like that, some days there might be a dozen, but they were always there. Most were just little stings, like those staples plucked from my neck in the hospital. But some readers were cruel and skilled. They'd slide the blade between my ribs in a way that would make me burn quiet tears at my desk. Once or twice I looked up a reader's address and fantasized about showing up at his front door. *I'm right here,* I'd say, fists already balled. *Say it to my face.*

I say all this knowing that in many ways I got off easy, because I'm a white guy. You don't want to see the emails the black women at the paper get.

To soothe the hurt I prowled the newsroom, scavenging for snacks. The *Observer* had some kind of party just about every day—a birthday or an award or a going-away for somebody leaving. Gary Wright, the court reporter, kept peanut butter crackers in his desk. There was always a bowl of M&M's around, or leftover Halloween candy. I'd bring a stash back to my cubicle, bandaging the cuts to my heart with tortilla chips or sheet cake. Sometimes I'd intend to use the snacks as rewards—make that difficult phone call and then have a cookie. But once the goods were laid out in front of me, I couldn't resist. Phone call, later. Sugar high, right fucking now.

There are lots of different ways to write a column. I tried to get out of the office, be a reporter, take on all the big stories. Sometimes that meant driving straight into darkness. I headed to Virginia Tech after the shootings there, the body count rising on the car radio as I drove toward Blacksburg and it started to snow. I covered the memorial in Charleston after nine firefighters died in a fire at a furniture store. I stood in a bare room at Central Prison in Raleigh after midnight, watching through a sheet of glass as a man who'd murdered his wife with a screwdriver died by lethal injection. My phone rang one January afternoon after a vice president at Wachovia Bank stabbed his twin five-year-old daughters to death. Every reporter in town was trying to find his wife. She called me.

I was drawn to those stories even as they kept me up at night. They felt like my duty. Readers, and editors, wanted me to try to make sense of the worst of the world. But I also wanted to sort it out for myself—not so much why people kill, or why the world can be so heartless, but how people deal with the pain. Being a fat guy was small and meaningless next to parents who had seen their children die. If I put myself in the middle of someone else's troubles, maybe I could find a way out of mine.

In 2005, the paper sent me to Louisiana to be part of a team writing about Hurricane Katrina. Every hotel was full so I slept in my rented SUV. I had covered several hurricanes and kept a duffel bag with the essentials: rain gear, flashlights, a radio, a good knife, toilet paper. Perishable food was no good—you couldn't count on power or ice—so I packed peanut butter, cans of Chef Boyardee, bottled water, and beer. Hundreds of reporters were in New Orleans so I veered south of the city to the bayous and the destroyed little fishing villages. I was driving on top of a levee one afternoon when I saw a man peek out of a ruined house. He had hidden in his attic with his dogs and cats when the hurricane came through. After we finished talking, I asked him if he wanted a beer. I had eighteen Budweisers left. Yes sir, he said, he wouldn't mind taking them all.

One morning I heard a rumor on the radio that twenty-two people in a little town called Violet had drowned together, lashed to one another by a rope. Violet is down in St. Bernard Parish, southeast of New Orleans. I drove around washed-out roadbeds and past packs of stray dogs to get down there. I asked if anybody knew about the people who died. *The sheriff did,* somebody said. *He just left.* I spent all day one step behind him, not able to reach him by phone, going deeper and deeper into wrecked country on flooded roads. A couple times I got to crossings where I couldn't see bottom. It was stupid to drive on. I drove on.

Late in the afternoon—I had driven at least a hundred miles by then—I made it to a shipyard where somebody told me the sheriff might be. A guy on the dock pointed me to a riverboat. I stepped onto the deck and found the sheriff in a vast ballroom, empty except for a deckhand pouring Diet Coke into the first ice I'd seen in days. It was like finding Colonel Kurtz on a cruise ship. I came in, unshowered and caked in mud, and told the sheriff what I was looking for. He hadn't seen the bodies but he confirmed the story. No other reporter was down here. Nobody else could possibly have it. It was a huge scoop.

The day was running out of light and it would take hours to backtrack. So I pushed ahead, looping back toward Baton Rouge, praying for unbroken roads until I could find electricity and cell service. After a while I ran into Interstate 10 east of the city. The road was empty, so I stopped the SUV in the median and got out to pee. Dozens of cars were abandoned on both shoulders. The land was flat and the horizon stretched out for miles in every direction. I was the only living creature I could see. There weren't even birds. I pissed on the highway and wondered if the rapture had happened and I was the one left behind to go to hell.

In a few miles I got to Lake Pontchartrain. About a mile across the bridge I slammed on the brakes—a section of the bridge was blown out. Now I was starting to panic. I didn't want to spend the night out there with whatever might come out of the swamp. I looked to the west and saw a second bridge running parallel. I doubled back, found the other highway, and crept out onto the second bridge. It was solid. I drove across the vast lake at ten miles an hour, alone.

On the other side, at the entrance to the town of Slidell, was a National Guardsman with a rifle. He quite reasonably wanted to know what the fuck I was doing out there. Slidell was blocked off and barricaded. But I told my story and he let me through with one instruction: *Don't stop*. I drove through slowly, looking at a whole town that Katrina had turned into toothpicks.

Back toward New Orleans, a few places had power. I made it to a Chinese restaurant and called my editor. By this time, I was starting to doubt the sheriff's story. I wanted to wait until we found somebody who had seen the bodies. The editor wanted to run the story—the sheriff had confirmed, and that was enough. We both knew it was a big story, we were both too tired to think straight, and I didn't have much fight left in me. I wrote the story on the hood of the SUV, taking what the sheriff had told me as fact.

You can probably guess how this ends. The sheriff had bad information. The whole story turned out to be false. We had to write a huge correction. Just about every piece looking back at Katrina mentions the Violet story as an example of how wild rumors ended up as actual news reports during the first days after the storm. I never should've written that story, especially at the end of that surreal day. Sometimes, in my dreams, I find myself stuck out on that empty highway, surrounded by abandoned cars, lost and alone.

My last night down there, they finally found me a place to sleep, with a group of LSU students who were renting a house in Baton Rouge. I knocked on the door and one of the guys let me in. There was a dog with him. The dog started growling. I looked toward the kitchen. There, in the doorway, was a goat.

The guy shook his head sadly. "That dog don't like that goat," he said.

I fell asleep in some student's bed with a pair of panties tacked to the wall, and wondered if the whole week had been a bad drug trip. I left the next morning, found some boudin and eggs, and pointed the SUV toward home. I was luckier than a lot of the people who had gone through Katrina. I had a home to head for.

I've made the job sound too bleak. Many days were a joy. I loved to write about the small kindnesses of life—one of my favorite columns was about a woman whose car died in the pouring rain in a mall parking lot, and how dozens of people stopped by to help. The writing gods brought gifts by the basketful. One day we found out that a loose group of amateur criminals had stolen seventeen million dollars from a Loomis Fargo armored car, then spent it on things like breast implants and a house with a velvet Elvis. The guy on the inside had fled to Mexico, where he hid out in a hotel eating M&M's and listening to "Hotel California." (All this ended up as a Zach Galifianakis movie called *Masterminds*, which was not nearly as good as the real story.) I was there in the courtroom when the tale first unfolded. "These folks are not exactly the brightest bulbs in the chandelier," I wrote, and that turned out to be accurate.

The best thing that happened was just a couple months after I took the columnist job. The *Observer* still had bureaus in smaller towns all around Charlotte. I wanted to know about those places, so I offered to visit each bureau, talk about writing, and swap some ideas. The bureau chief in Hickory, an hour north of Charlotte, was a friendly and sharp editor from Wisconsin named Alix Felsing. She wanted me to talk to the staff and give her some writing advice—she was getting ready to leave for a new job at the paper in Columbia, South Carolina, and was working on her farewell column.

Alix and I had both started at the *Observer* in 1989, eight years before, but we'd never worked in the same office. We'd see each other at the Mothership every so often, or bump into each other at a party once or twice a year. I always figured she had a boyfriend, and I found out later that she always figured I had a girlfriend. When we started talking, there in the bureau in Hickory, I could tell right away that I'd missed out on someone special. She touched all four bases that mattered most to me—she was funny, smart, sexy, and kind. After I talked to the staff, we went into her office to talk about her farewell column. She mentioned she was going to the Hickory Crawdads minor league baseball game that night. Would I like to go and talk some more? Absolutely. She changed into shorts and I noticed she also had great legs. I snuck looks the whole game through my sunglasses.

We did not consider this a date. Everybody in her office considered it a date.

That weekend, I took her to a party at our friend Dan Huntley's house on the lake so she could say goodbye to friends. We did not consider this a date. Everybody there considered it a date. We hugged hard at the end of the night. She was moving ninety miles away. Best not to think about her. I kept thinking about her.

She wrote me a note thanking me for the company. I turned the note over and over in my hands, thought about whether I should say what I really wanted to say. I'd dated around, had a couple of girlfriends, but most of the time, when I really wanted someone, they didn't want me back. And to be honest, looking at myself in the mirror, I figured they were making a good call.

But I couldn't stop thinking about Alix. I wrote back and told her how I felt. She wrote back and said she felt the same. We arranged for me to stop by her house in Columbia on the way back from a reporting trip to Florida. She opened the door and I kissed her. A thunderstorm came in the night and hail bounced on her front lawn. *That* was our first date. It was the summer of 1997. We've been together since.

The first trip we took together was just a few weeks later—a flight to Wisconsin to meet her extended family on their yearly camping trip. It was the first time I ate sauerbraten. I'm pretty sure it was the first time I had *seen* sauerbraten. One afternoon Alix and I went for a long walk in the woods. After a couple of miles I felt a familiar sting in my right thigh. It comes from my gut pressing down on the nerves at the top of my leg. My doctor calls it a gunslinger— people used to get it in the old West from the weight of the guns on their belts. The pinched nerves set my leg on fire. We stopped and sat on a low stone wall.

"You need to know," I said. "I'm damaged goods."

By then I was thirty-three and weighed more than four hundred pounds. Alix was in great shape and went running just about every day in the South Carolina heat. I was falling hard for her. I could feel her falling for me. But I couldn't understand how. All I could see was the disgusting man all those readers wrote about. Never had I felt like any woman I'd ever dated was going to stay. Alix felt like she might stay. I needed to warn her.

"I'm damaged goods," I said again.

"No, you're not," she said.

On the flight back home she slept with her head on my shoulder. I didn't tell her I loved her until later. But I loved her right then.

We got engaged six months after we started dating, and got married six months after we got engaged. I wrote a column that ran on our wedding day. People still come up to me on the street and talk about it. Some of them keep it in their pocketbooks. Others have passed it to their children. There's a special joy that comes out of loneliness rescued by love. I know Alix rescued me. Here's the column:

Unless I screw up between now and "I will," sometime around 6:30 this evening I will become a married man.

Little problems mean nothing today. If I lose the rings we'll use tinfoil. If I forget my tux I'll go naked. If I have a flat tire I'll jog to the service, and my bride-to-be knows how much I hate jogging.

Alexandra Dawn Felsing (she goes by Alix) knows a lot of other things about me. She knows I like to stack my towels in an alternating pattern, colored, white, colored, white. She knows I wiggle my right foot when I get excited, like a dog getting his belly rubbed. She knows I cry more than the average guy.

I know things about her, too. I know how her eyes light up when she finds a cool piece of fabric at Mary Jo's in Gastonia. I know how she ditched piano lessons as a kid to go outside and play softball. I know how she likes her privacy and is probably getting twitchy just thinking about these words on the page.

We are opposites in so many ways. I'm from Georgia, she's from Wisconsin. I like bright shiny colors, she likes browns and greens. I like music, she likes Neil Diamond.

But we have lots in common, too. We think the Lord invented summer nights for minor league baseball, and created newspapers as a place to put the comic strips.

Lately we also have the habit of just staring at each other, amazed that all this is really happening, astonished that the fullness in our hearts is not a trick of nature or a fleeting attraction but the soft steady drumbeat of love.

I always hoped I would find someone and we would fall in love. But I didn't think I had much to offer, especially in those first few moments where you make an impression or you slink back across the room. I came to believe I was just a fat guy with bad teeth, and I pretty much quit trying.

The only reason my heart didn't get broken is because I rarely took it out of the box.

Alix and I had both worked here at the *Observer* for years, but the paper has offices in several towns and we never worked in the same place. Last summer I found out she was moving away. I knew her just well enough to want to say goodbye.

I visited her office in Hickory. We went to a ball game that night, then a party that weekend. Then she left town. And I couldn't stop thinking about her.

Still, I planned to let it go. Long-distance romances don't work, that's what I told myself. But what I really believed was: She's out of my league.

But a few days later she sent me a thank-you note. It took me two days to muster the guts to write back. I filled the letter with escape hatches and exit doors, giving her every chance to let me down easy. But somehow I sputtered out that I had been thinking romantic thoughts about her.

A couple of days later I got a note from her, saying she had been thinking the same thing. I got up off the floor and called her.

And here we are.

I don't pretend to know how love works. I can tell you a thousand things I love about Alix, but none of them are exactly why I love her. The why, I don't have words for. It's a code we decipher every time we hold hands, a secret song we hear when we look in each other's eyes.

It's really true. You just know.

The point of this is not to brag about my good fortune. It is simply to say that no matter how lonely you are, no matter how much you think you've missed your chance, there is hope, always hope, everlasting hope.

Today my fondest hopes come true. And sometime around 6:30 this evening, I'll become the luckiest man alive.

On our wedding day, as I squeezed into my rented tux, I promised myself that I'd earn the trust Alix put in me. We committed for better or worse, but to hell with worse. I'd get in shape. We'd run together. We talked about it on long car rides and on slow Sunday mornings with our legs tangled together on the couch. Every young married couple dreams. Those were our dreams. They depended on me doing something I had never been able to do.

In 2008, I hit the professional lottery—I was chosen for a Nieman Fellowship at Harvard. It's designed for midcareer journalists who need a break and want to study something in depth. You get a full school year away from work to audit classes, go to lectures and concerts, hang out on the Harvard campus, and make new friends from around the world. Plus, they pay you. It's ridiculous.

A few weeks before we left for Cambridge, I stopped by my doctor's office for a physical. Part of the physical was an ultrasound of my heart, a routine procedure for someone my size. (Even though I've always been fat, I've never had a hint of heart trouble.) I was lying on my side on the examining table when the guy doing the ultrasound said "Hmmm."

You never want anybody giving you a medical exam to say "Hmmm."

He went to get my doctor, Al Hudson. They said "Hmmm." Dr. Hudson called in a heart doctor who worked in the same building. They all said "Hmmm." I did not think *Hmmm*. I thought *Oh, shit*.

They consulted briefly and nodded in agreement. Then Dr. Hudson told me I had a tumor in my heart.

It's called an atrial myxoma. Google it sometime. You can even find video. It's a benign tumor that grows inside one of the chambers of the heart—usually the left atrium. It's held in there by a little tether of tissue, like a balloon on a string. The tumor wasn't causing any damage—nobody knew it was there before the ultrasound. But it was taking up a lot of room in the atrium. The doctors said it could shift and plug the atrial valve, or break loose and cause a blood clot. Either of those things could kill me. The rule among doctors is, once you know it's in there, it has to come out.

Dr. Hudson was excited. I was the first atrial myxoma he'd ever had.

I was not excited. Especially when they said the words *open heart surgery*.

Everybody assured me this particular type of open heart surgery was no big deal. The surgeon would be inside my heart for just a few minutes, long enough to snip out the tumor. The hardest part would be cutting open my chest.

I was also not excited at the words *cutting open my chest*.

It had been eleven years since Alix and I got married, and I had made all those promises to her to get in better shape. I hadn't kept a single one. I'd do OK for a while—take long walks, shoot some hoops, eat more broccoli—but before long I'd backslide. Now I had to tell her about this. I called her at work and asked her to meet me in the parking lot under the building. I drew the little diagram of my heart, the same way Dr. Kamerer had drawn the little diagram of my voice box fifteen years before. We sat there in the car, too stunned to say much, knowing the words underneath the words: Even if the surgery itself wasn't dangerous, I made it dangerous because I was still so fat.

I asked the anesthesiologist about it. "Yeah, it would be easier if you were two hundred pounds lighter," he said. Not reassuring. I was OK until the night before the surgery, trying to sleep in the hospital room, worried that my weight would cause a crisis on the operating table and I would die there, having finally fucked up for good. I started crying and couldn't stop. Alix crawled into the hospital bed next to me.

I woke up in a recovery room just like the one I'd woken up in fifteen years before. Instead of the slash in my neck, there was a column of stitches down the middle of my chest.

The doctors were right—the surgery went fine. I was up and moving around right away. I went home a couple days later. We have so many good friends and neighbors, and they brought comfort food. Two friends from church brought a shepherd's pie big enough to feed every shepherd in Europe. It tasted so good. I wasn't on any dietary restrictions from the surgery. I pulled the same old con on my brain—it's just one meal, you deserve it, you can get in shape later. I piled it in, putting more work on my newly scarred heart.

I had pretty much healed by the time the fellowship started. Harvard was good for my soul and, it turned out, my body. Alix and I lived a half mile from Harvard Yard and we walked everywhere—three or four miles a day to classes and concerts and movies and parties, plus walking Fred two or three times a day. The fellowship provided lots of free food and Sam Adams. I learned to love sushi, which they fed us almost every Friday. I ate a tankful of lobsters. Still, I lost twenty pounds and felt as good as I had in years. Our tribe was large—twenty-five fellows, plus spouses and kids and the Nieman staff—and our friendships deepened over walks in the snow and long nights of drinking and talking and decoding the mysteries of the world.

Each fellow has one night during the year called a sounding, where you basically tell your life story. Everybody eats a meal you provide. We found a place in Boston that had a pretty good take on North Carolina barbecue. We made two special Southern dishes ourselves—pimento cheese and banana pudding. I put a sign next to the pimento cheese:

SPREAD OF THE GODS

CHEESE + MAYO + PIMENTOS + OLIVES = HEALTH FOOD!*

*MAY KILL YOU

We also made banana pudding the way I remembered it from home—layers of sliced bananas, vanilla pudding, vanilla wafers, and whipped cream. Apparently banana pudding is not something they serve in the far reaches of the globe. "WHAT IS THIS?" our Russian friend Andrei said after his first bite, as though his spoon had unearthed a vein of diamonds. Every scrap was gone by the end of the night. There were other big meals at the soundings, but ours won the prize for the highest calorie count. Where I come from, it was just an ordinary Sunday supper. I felt like

Mama feels when she has our big family over for a meal—like I was sharing the most valuable treasures we had. There has never been better food created anywhere than the food of the American South. There has never been any food that will make you fatter. Sometimes I wonder if I'd still be fat if I had been born in Sweden or Ecuador or anywhere else but the bottom right corner of the USA. It's one of those unanswerable questions they talk about in philosophy class. Nature vs. nurture. Man vs. pimento cheese.

We got back from Harvard in 2009 and I wanted to try new things at the paper—blogging, longer features, maybe some sportswriting. Being a columnist is in some ways like being in a popular band. Some of your fans love it when you veer off in other directions, but most of them want you to keep playing the hits, because that's why they became fans in the first place. It has always been important to me to work hard no matter what—being a professional means doing the job even on days when you don't feel like it. But after a year or two back at the paper, I was drifting. My creative energy for columns was tapped out. I turned into the type of reporter who used to piss me off—staying in the office, missing deadlines, moping at my desk. I hit the snack tables at work even harder. Sometimes that wasn't enough and I'd go downstairs to the vending machines. I'd buy a pack of Ruffles and three candy bars and stuff it all in my pockets so nobody could see my gluttony. I'd try not to get caught in any long conversations on the way back to my desk. If I lingered, my body heat would melt my Snickers.

My career changed with a single story. I had been doing a little freelancing on the side so I could write different kinds of stories and make a little extra money. In early 2011, I couldn't stop reading about a bizarre tale out of Alabama. The Alabama-Auburn football rivalry is the most hateful feud in American sports. In 2010, Auburn quarterback Cam Newton (now an NFL star with the Carolina Panthers) led a huge comeback to beat Alabama—the Tigers were down 24–0 and came back to win 28–27. That night, a crazed Alabama fan named Harvey Updyke drove to the Auburn campus. At the entrance to the campus were two ancient oak trees called Toomer's Oaks. The trees symbolized Auburn—old college friends reunited there, and legions of Auburn men had proposed under the oaks. They were also the spot where fans gathered after a big sports win. Fans would roll the oaks with toilet paper whenever Auburn won a big game. Harvey Updyke hated Auburn and so he hated Toomer's Oaks. In the middle of the night, he slipped into Toomer's Corner, where the oaks stood, and poured poison on the two trees—enough to kill an acre of brush. Nobody knew he had done it until months later, when he called in to the Paul Finebaum radio show and bragged about it. By then it was too late for the trees. They were going to die.

College football is the sport I love most. I have spent my whole life watching SEC football. I understand what Alabama-Auburn means to that state, how the rivalry burns like a bonfire all year long, how that heat creates somebody like Harvey Updyke. I could hear the story's heartbeat. Joe Posnanski, my friend from the *Observer* bureaus, had landed at *Sports Illustrated*. He connected me with his editor, Chris Stone. I pitched the story, and when Chris hesitated, I took vacation time to drive to Auburn and do reporting on my own dime. Chris bought the story. I wrote it on nights and weekends after getting home from the paper. It ended up making that year's edition of *The Best American Sports Writing*. It also gave me the creative juice I'd been missing at the office. It felt like the next step I'd been waiting to take.

A few months later, in 2012, Joe took a job as the first writer for a start-up site called Sports on Earth. He recommended me, and they offered me a job. I had been at the *Observer* for twenty-three years, and I felt guilty for wanting to leave. The paper tried to keep me. But I didn't want to get to retirement never having tried something new, wondering what I'd missed. They threw a big going-away party. I gave a little speech and said something I still believe: When you write for the paper—or when you create anything, really—you make yourself immortal. In our business, the place where they store old clip files is called the morgue. But really, it's the opposite. It's where we live forever.

A few years ago, when newspapers started shedding employees, the *Observer* started a beautiful tradition. On your last day, when you walk out, everybody in the office stands and applauds. So on my last day, I had one last plate of newsroom food, sent out a farewell note, grabbed the box of stuff I had cleaned out of my desk, and left with Alix to a standing ovation.

I should have been the one applauding them.

I still miss writing for the paper, but more than that I miss just coming to the office every day and shooting the shit with all the funny and smart and weird and fantastic people who make up a newsroom. I've felt like an outsider my whole life. I've never felt more like I belonged somewhere than I did in that newsroom. And, yeah, I miss the free cheese cubes.

Sports on Earth struggled to find readers and make money. Most start-ups fail in one way or another. I knew the risk when I took the job. A year and four months after I started, they fired me, and pretty soon they fired just about everybody else. It stuck around a few more years, a sliver of what it was, and a sliver of a sliver of what we hoped it would be. But I'll always be glad for the chance.

Since then I've been a freelancer, working from my home office or a coffee shop or a hotel room somewhere. I've spent so much of my life staring at a blank page, looking for the right words. Almost all of them have been about other people. It's weird to be writing about myself. Part of the magic of writing is that it helps you discover what you think. Here's what I've discovered so far, by writing all this down: I've had a good life. But it would have been so much better, at every step, if I hadn't been dragging all this extra weight around.

Being fat made me a kid who turned inward. Being fat made me stand out to people inclined to be cruel. Being fat made me think I'd never find love. Being fat made me doubt every good thing about myself.

Being fat made me.

The past tense is wrong there, I know. I'm still fat, so it still makes me what I am. But part of what I'm trying to do is drag the past back into the past. From here on out, I have to unmake me.

MARCH

It's Pi Day—3.14.15—so we go looking for pie.

Alix and I aren't much for big celebrations. We did each other right on our fiftieth birthdays—I got her best friends to come from out of town on hers, and she threw a surprise party with a houseful of friends for mine. But other than that we're low-key. Christmas is a book or tickets to a show. We're just not big on stuff. Instead we have a lot of little celebrations. Pi Day is one of those little nerdy things we love.

So we head to our favorite diner in Charlotte, a place called the Landmark. Guy Fieri's face is spray-painted on the wall—he came here a few years ago for *Diners, Drive-ins and Dives*. (As you might imagine, Triple D is one of my favorite shows.) The 2:00 a.m. people-watching at the Landmark is unparalleled. Sometimes you'll get a church choir in one corner and a bunch of bikers in another. When we go there, we usually get a late breakfast—eggs and bacon or pancakes. But like most classic diners, they have a giant display case of sweets just inside the door. The layer cakes and cinnamon rolls pull like a tractor beam. On Pi Day we let ourselves be sucked in.

Alix gets key lime. I get banana cream. Each slice could feed an orphanage. I cut through the whipped cream on my slice and hit something solid. It turns out there's an entire banana hidden along the outer rim. We wash it all down with coffee and fall straight into a sugar coma.

We are actually celebrating something more than Pi Day. After months of thinking about it—and not quite three years after I quit the *Observer*—Alix put in her notice at the publishing center where she did copyediting and design for the *Observer* and two other papers. They were getting ready to let go twenty percent of the staff, and the severance was pretty good, so she raised her hand to be laid off. She struggled with leaving the same way I did. Newspaper life is about all we've ever known. But she has spent the last four years taking classes at night and getting her master's in organizational development. As part of that, she earned a certificate to be an executive coach. She wants to use those skills in new ways. It's a big leap for her and for us. For nearly all our adult lives, we've had steady salaried jobs with benefits. Now neither one of us has a full-time gig.

Part of making this work, we agree, is cutting expenses. Our biggest expense besides the bills we have to pay is going out to eat. When we go out with friends, it's worth it for the experience and the good company. But too often we go out when we're tired or brain-fried or bored with whatever's in the fridge. The whole concept of a restaurant is comforting. *Just sit right here, honey. We'll bring you something good.*

The other thing is, restaurants are willing to do things that you would never do yourself. "You know why restaurant food is so good?" our buddy Dan Huntley, a journalist turned caterer and barbecue god, told us one night. "Ghee." Ghee is clarified butter—like butter concentrate. Put enough ghee in the pan and you could make an old shoe taste good. Restaurants use big chunks of ghee, or shit-tons of regular butter. Some places fry stuff in lard. Just about every place uses a heavy hand with salt and sugar and cream. And you pay them to do it.

At home we'd never make a banana cream pie to begin with, much less one with a whole banana in each slice. But at the Landmark, on Pi Day, somehow it makes sense. Pi, as far as we know, has an infinite number of digits. Pie, we know for sure, has a tremendous number of calories. My best guess, after consulting with my Fitbit guide, is that my slice of banana cream had 700. I can almost hear my little black wristband going *noooooooooo*.

We know better than to celebrate the big moments in our lives with food. We know better than to go out to eat so much. It's bad for both of us. But it's hard for us to tear away from tradition. It's as tasty and seductive as a mouthful of pie.

Weight on February 28: 452

Weight on March 31: 456

For the month: +4

For the year: -4

Four

GREASE IS THE WORD

I cheat on my wife with a redhead named Wendy. Her place is just a couple of miles from our house. She's always smiling when I pull up. She gives me exactly what I want. Every time I leave, I swear I won't come back. I keep coming back.

Wendy is my favorite, but she's not my only one. Sometimes I go across town for a quickie with a guy in a clown suit named Ronald.

Fast food is my deepest addiction. Since I was sixteen and got my first car, I've spent endless hours idling in drive-through lanes, waiting to trade my money for my fix. I did some deeply depressing calculations one afternoon and figured out that I've spent at least thirty dollars a week on fast food for the last thirty-five years. That comes to somewhere around fifty-five thousand dollars. Fuuuuuck. That's enough for a bass boat or a new kitchen, with some left over to stash in the bank. Instead, I have invested it in Big Macs and big pants. If you're addicted to anything and want to get one solid measure of how much it has hurt your life: Do the math.

Next time you go to a fast-food joint, take a slow walk around the parking lot. You'll find the spaces filled with customers eating in their cars. That's where the junkies hang out. Alone in your car, you can get the double Whopper *and* the onion rings *and* the chocolate shake, and nobody knows but the cashier who hands you the bag. Every car I've owned has ended up with salt in the cracks of the passenger seat and leftover napkins in the glove box.

It always makes me laugh to hear people say fast food doesn't taste good. They are obviously trying to convince themselves. Fast food tastes FANTASTIC. It has been engineered and test-marketed and focus-grouped by billion-dollar corporations whose profits depend on getting customers to come back. God knows what meatish substance they use to fill a Taco Bell taco, but it's amazing. On the face of it, a Big Mac is a terrible bargain. It's ninety percent bread and shredded lettuce. Somewhere deep inside are two little disks of meat. But once you spelunk your way in there, those last three bites are fucking awesome. Eating a Big Mac is like being a shitty golfer. You might shoot 120, but all you remember is that one drive that split the middle of the fairway.

The main object of my food lust is a Wendy's double with cheese: two greasy beef patties, sandwiched around a slice of American, nestled in a soft white bun. Foodies talk about umami, that sixth sense of food where savory flavor and tongue-coating texture blend into something damn near erotic. I get my Wendy's double all the way, but the part I really like is out on the edge, where the meat and the cheese and the bread melt into pure umami. It's a burst of pleasure so powerful I want it again and again.

Not long ago, I was in the drive-through and called out my regular order.

"I'll have a number two combo, medium-sized, with a Dr Pepper, and—"

The cashier cut in.

"—And a junior bacon, right?"

"Right."

Wait, what?

Shit.

I was at the anonymous fast-food joint, ordering in the most anonymous way possible. But I went there so often that the cashier knew what I wanted just from my voice.

I'd become a regular.

I told myself I was never going back again.

I was back in a week.

By the way: My regular order (double cheese combo with medium fries and Dr Pepper, plus a junior bacon cheeseburger) costs $10.37 at my local Wendy's. But that's not the real price. The FDA says the average American man should eat about 2,500 calories a day. That meal alone comes in at 1,910.

Burger King was a big night for us when I was a kid. In the 1970s, the three of us could eat for less than ten bucks. My mom and dad made minimum wage, or somewhere around it, for most of their lives. The local Sizzler might as well have been the Four Seasons. It's easy to look down on fast food. But it's a cheap night out of the house, and when you're poor, that counts for a lot.

Still, we mostly ate at home. I didn't start scarfing fast food in volume until I was in high school, working at the drive-in, making my own money. My friend Bert, who ran the projectors, lived his life in exclamation points. He did pull-ups on the metal beams at the concession stand. He hit massive home runs in our Saturday softball games. He wired home stereo speakers to the tape deck in his station wagon and blasted "Bohemian Rhapsody." He ate big, too, and spent a lot of time thinking about how to get the maximum fast food for his money. He had decided the best deal was regular cheeseburgers at McDonald's. So once a week, after softball, we'd hit the drive-through and split a dozen. I was fourteen years old but felt grown and rich. Every time that bag came through the window, it looked like a sack of doubloons.

When I got my own car, my fast-food intake quintupled. Maybe it heptupled or octupled. There was definitely tupling going on. McDonald's on the way home from school. Steak tacos from Del Taco on the way back from the beach. In those days I played a lot of tennis with my best friends Virgil and Perry. After the match we'd hydrate with vodka and Gatorade. Then I'd grab a sack of Krystal burgers on the way home. I believe this was also John McEnroe's fitness program in the eighties.

The great writer Calvin Trillin once said that if you don't think your hometown hamburger place is the best hamburger place in the world, you're a sissy. In that spirit, let me inform you that my hometown hot-dog joint, Willie's Wee-Nee Wagon, is the best hot-dog joint in the world. I would argue (and have argued) that it is the best *restaurant* in the world. It's a homely old low-slung building on Altama Avenue, the main drag in Brunswick. There's an awning, a screened-in porch, and a few picnic tables. The paint and the light are both yellowish. The sign out front reads WE RELISH YOUR BUN.

Willie's makes great greasy burgers and pork chop sandwiches, but I never have those, because their hot dogs strike me directly in the soul. They're perfectly grilled, cradled in steamed sesame-seed buns, with steak fries on the side and tea so sweet it could hold its shape without a cup. You can get a dog a dozen different ways at Willie's, but I always default to a simple dog with coleslaw and cheese. I did a travel story on my hometown for the *Charlotte Observer* back in the nineties and wrote that if I were ever elected president, I'd have slaw-and-cheese dogs from Willie's delivered to the White House every day. Somebody from Willie's saw the story, clipped out that paragraph, and hung it on the wall. Twenty-some years later, it's still there. This is one of my proudest achievements.

Everybody needs a third place—a bar or a coffee shop or a bookstore—somewhere to feel comfortable that's not work or home. Willie's was my third place for a lot of years. I went there to meet old friends. I went after getting in trouble with my folks. I took dates there at the end of the night, when our clothes were tousled and our appetites high. I slunk back there after getting dumped. I went when I didn't know what else to do. I'd sit on the hood of my car, and somebody I knew would eventually show up.

A couple weeks after my sister died, I drove the forty miles from her place in Jesup to Willie's. I ordered a dog and some fries and a tea and sat at one of the picnic tables to wait. The aroma sunk into my bones. The flow of customers coming up to the window was as familiar as breathing. They called out my order. I ate in the car. I grieved for Brenda and felt a little better.

This sounds pathetic, I know, but one of the things I get from fast food is companionship. I'm an introvert who learned to talk to strangers because I love my work and how it makes me feel. I adore my wife and family and friends. But I spent so much time alone in my room growing up. So much time alone when I was single. So much time working a day shift while Alix worked nights. These days I spend so much time working at home or in a hotel room somewhere. Aloneness has become my natural state. That's not who I want to be, but it's who I am. I have lived most of my life in my mind.

On those days when the gravity of solitude tries to pin me down, fast food serves as a little bridge to the other side. Sometimes, when I'm in a creative rut, I'll take a drive to get out of the house and see things with a fresh eye. Almost always, I'll end up in a drive-through somewhere. Maybe I'll sit in the car and people-watch. Maybe I'll just take my food home. But at least, I tell myself, I've been out among people for a while. I've tried to be human.

This is the cruel trick of most addictions. They're so good at short-term comfort. I'm hungry, I'm lonely, I need to feel a part of the world. Other people soothe those pains with the bottle or the needle. I soothe them with burgers and fries. It pushes the hurt down the road a little bit, like paying the minimum on your credit-card bill every month. The debt never gets settled. Those little moments of comfort are also moments of avoiding the discomfort behind it. In that small instant when the salt and grease get into my veins, it's a release. But then, when I look up and out and back, my life is measured not in days or years or heartbeats but in an unbroken string of takeout bags.

Fast food is not just burgers and tacos. It's the stuff in vending machines and Jiffy Marts and the quick-foods aisle at the grocery store—all that stuff processed to the point where you're not sure exactly what it's made of. (I've eaten a million Cheetos in my life, but until I looked it up the other day, I never knew what the base ingredient was. Cornmeal, it turns out. There's not a single thing about a Cheeto that makes me think of corn.)

The convenience store where I buy gas has a big rack of candy bars just inside the front door. At the top it has a photo of various snacks—M&M's and gummy bears and mixed nuts, all arranged in mounds. The advertising pitch is just eight words:

SWEET CHEWY SOUR SALTY
The Flavors You Crave

You have to admire the copywriter who came up with that. There's nothing subtle about it. There's no half-hearted nod toward nutrition. It's not even about what you *like*. It's about what you *crave*. Convenience stores are places where people make thousands of bad decisions every day—lottery tickets, malt liquor, Marlboro reds, taquitos that have been spinning on that rolling warmer for two or three years. Some convenience stores sell wine in *individual glasses*, with *lids*, just in case you need a few slugs of chardonnay to get through the drive home. But nothing else in the store is advertised with the bluntness of junk food. There's no sign over the cigarette rack that says NICOTINE—THE CHEMICAL YOU CRAVE.

I'm hooked on junk food in much the same way I'm hooked on football. Every Saturday and Sunday I watch players get carted off the field with concussions and shredded ACLs, but I try hard not to think about it because the game is so brutally beautiful. The difference with junk food is, it's tearing up my *own* body. The evidence is obvious. But I'm so drawn to it that I'm not sure how far the junk-food giants would have to go to make me quit.

We're now making Cheez-Its from cat hair and sawdust. Deal with it.

All right, dammit. Gimme the party-sized box.

Just look at what they've done to potatoes. A plain potato, baked or boiled, is not terrible for you. It's not exactly health food, but it has vitamins and fiber. Potatoes kept Matt Damon alive in *The Martian*. He wouldn't have survived on beets.

But dip potatoes in grease and they can kill you a hundred different ways, all of which I love. Waffle House hash browns, scattered on the grill and smothered with onions. Home fries, spread out in chunks next to a three-egg omelet. Tater tots, better out of the frozen-food aisle than at any restaurant. Bo-tato Rounds, the garlicky hockey pucks made by Bojangles', the Southern fried-chicken chain. I could eat a stack of Bo-tato Rounds as high as my head.

French fries might be the one and only thing every American loves—we eat nearly thirty pounds per person per year. Picky little kids eat them. Old folks with weak stomachs eat them. Vegetarians and carnivores eat them. People who claim to hate fast food put on shades and a hat so they won't get caught in the line for fries at McDonald's. My wife, being virtuous, almost never orders fries. She just sneaks them off my plate. *They need to be tested,* she says.

But to me, the pinnacle of potato evolution is the potato chip. Other fried potatoes balance soft innards with a crispy crust. Potato chips are all crust. They don't even taste that much like potatoes— they're salt and grease and whatever magic dust they're coated with. It seems as if every week there are new flavors: sriracha, ketchup, biscuits and gravy. They've yet to make one I don't like. My favorite chips in the world are Utz sour cream and onion ripple chips. That green-and-white bag sways in my mind like a hula dancer. I've been staying away from them, trying to cut at least one thing out of my junk-food diet, but the ghost of the taste is still on my tongue. Every time I go in the grocery store, they're buy one, get one free. *He's been holding out,* says the store manager in my daydream, twirling his mustache. *But he still wants them. Oh yes he does.*

My worst fast-food spirals happen when Alix is out of town. Some days I'll wake up and grab sausage biscuits and Bo-tato Rounds for breakfast, then a Big Mac meal for lunch, then my regular Wendy's for supper. Sub in a big bag of Utz for the fries. Add a sleeve of Chips Ahoy or a pint of Ben & Jerry's for dessert.

I did the math on all this one day and it just about knocked me over. On a really bad day I might eat 6,000 calories—roughly the same amount as the daily consumption for the average adult tiger. And it goes without saying that I'm not spending half my day chasing down wildebeest.

How does a human being end up weighing 460 pounds? Six thousand calories at a time.

I've never done hard drugs, but on the worst days I feel the way I've always imagined a heroin addict feels—blissful on the outside, self-hating underneath, chained to an anchor in a bottomless ocean. No way to make it to the surface. Might as well let go.

This is where the discussion about obesity always ends up: temptation vs. free will.

In some ways, human self-control is no match for the junk-food industry. The big food companies push sugary cereals and nutrition-free snacks to kids from the time they're old enough to stare at a TV screen. (I can still sing the Honeycomb cereal theme from the seventies commercials—*Honeycomb's big / Yeah yeah yeah / It's not small / No no no*—even though I'm pretty sure I never ate a mouthful of Honeycomb cereal.) It feels wrongheaded at best, and evil at worst, for companies to put so much money and skill into making people want food that can ruin and kill them. In his awful life, Pablo Escobar never sold a product that hooked as many people as Oreos.

But the libertarian in me (it's a small area near my gallbladder) believes that dodging the threats of the world is my own responsibility—especially as an adult. I wish constant sleepless nights on the advertising execs who get kids hooked on junk food. But what they made me crave when I was six shouldn't dictate my life today. In the same way, all that fried chicken I ate growing up doesn't make my mom and dad responsible for the Popeyes I ate yesterday. They did the best they knew how. I ought to do the best I know how. At some point we have to own our choices. If not, we're eternally children.

For the last few years, every time I've bought fast food, I've kept the receipt in my billfold. The idea is that one of those meals will be the last fast-food meal I ever eat, and I want the receipt as a reminder. For now it's a weary ritual: I buy something from the drive-through, toss the old receipt from my last meal, and replace it with the newest mistake. At my worst, I swap it out twice a day. For me, the biggest step toward becoming healthier is to just stop eating crap. It also feels like the hardest step.

Every so often I pull out the latest receipt and look at it. Most days the ink is still fresh. I think about that day when I'll pull one out and it'll be so old that it's yellowed and faded. I think about the day when it won't be a symbol anymore but just a useless scrap of paper. I think about the day when I can throw it in the trash, not needing the reminder anymore, because I broke the addiction before it broke me.

APRIL

My mom hates to go to the doctor. She'll walk around half dead before she breaks down and calls for an appointment. Her logic makes perfect crazy sense: When you go to the doctor, they always find something wrong with you. I get on her all the time about it. But the truth is, I'm the same way. I know I need a checkup here in the first part of the year to make sure I don't have any other serious problems as I start losing weight. But I keep putting it off. When I finally make the call, they inform me I haven't been in *four years*. Like mama, like son.

Thing is, I love our doctor. Dr. Hudson took care of Alix before we got married, and he took me on as a patient afterward. He's about our age, but most of his patients are in their seventies or eighties. "Thank you for being the youngest person I'll see all day!" he always says to Alix and me. "You might have a problem I can actually fix!" He's kind, generous, brilliant. But I'm still afraid to see him, because I know just how deep a hole I've dug. I'm worried he'll tell me it's too late to climb out.

I stop by to give blood for some tests. They have to draw the blood from the veins in my hands—there's too much fat in my arms for them to find the normal vein in the crook of my elbow. One time, when I was in the hospital, they couldn't get enough from my hands and had to jab the needle into the top of my foot. It's what made me quit giving blood years ago—not the pain, but the embarrassment—even though I'm O-negative, a blood type hospitals always need.

A few days later, I come back for a checkup and full report. Somehow I'm in decent shape for someone in terrible shape. My blood pressure is a tad high—140 over 90—but not dangerous. My cholesterol is in the normal range. I don't show any signs of diabetes, which is astounding given the amount of sugar I've shoveled in over my lifetime. I'm always surprised when my blood work comes back and I'm not wheeled straight to the ER. I think of my body like that car in *The Blues Brothers*—I've abused it so much that one day it'll just collapse in a heap of spare parts. Lots of people my age have to take regular medications for one thing or another. The only pills I take are vitamins and the occasional Tylenol. I'm skating on luck and good genes.

Dr. Hudson is thrilled that I'm finally losing weight, even though it's coming off slow. He says ninety-one percent of people who are overweight end up getting larger instead of smaller. To be in the nine percent, even if I've lost just a little bit of weight, is a big deal.

A few days later, I come back to interview Dr. Hudson about obesity. It's the main disease he treats. He doesn't think of treating obesity—or most other medical problems—as being about drugs or surgery. It's mostly about habits.

"When we talk about health-care reform, it's not really health-care reform," he says. "The Affordable Care Act and all that stuff—that's just about who pays. If we can get people to not smoke, to drink just a little and eat better—that's health-care reform."

Heart disease is the most obvious issue for fat people. When I had my atrial myxoma a few years ago, they did a cardiac catheterization as part of the prep. Everything looked clear, but as Dr. Hudson says, in a third of heart disease cases, the first symptom is death. That's not comforting.

Diabetes is the next worry. But cancer is also an issue. He says studies have linked at least four cancers—breast, lung, prostate, and colon—to excess weight. Statistically speaking, my throat cancer from twenty-two years ago doesn't make me any more likely to have cancer again. But it's always in the back of my mind. Once you've been hit by a car, it's hard not to think about being hit by another car.

The day I went to get my blood tests, they asked me to skip lunch so it wouldn't affect the readings. I got out of there around four and I hadn't eaten since eight in the morning. I got in the car and went straight to Wendy's.

But that was one dumb decision. I made a lot of better ones this month. I took a walk just about every day. Most days I avoided the drive-through. I'm hanging tough in the nine percent. It feels so good to be out of the ninety-one.

Weight on March 31: 456

Weight on April 30: 454

For the month: -2

For the year: -6

Five

A BODY AT REST

Every body perseveres in its state of rest, or of uniform motion
in a right line, unless it is compelled to change that state by
forces impressed thereon.

–Isaac Newton's first law of motion

T his will be as close as I ever get to bragging about my body:
I'm seventy-three inches tall, and the top six inches are sexy
as hell. My eyes are Paul Newman blue. My hair is congressional
quality. Everything from the bridge of my nose north has treated
me pretty well.

From there down, I'm a Superfund site.

I almost never get eight hours of sleep because my back starts
to hurt—Dr. Hudson says there's probably a little tear in one of the
disks. That pain goes away as soon as I get up and move around a
little. But I'm too big to just hop up. Here's the launch sequence I
follow to get out of bed: First I roll onto my right side. I dig my right
elbow into the mattress and hook my right leg over the edge of the
bed. Then I push with the elbow and pull with the leg until I'm sitting up. I stand up slow and straight, because if I twist I could hurt

my back even worse. (I throw out my back once a year or so, always doing some ordinary thing like tying my shoelaces or bending in the shower. I did it one time reaching for a fork in the silverware drawer. I've never quite understood the definition of *irony*, but I think that might be it.)

Finally, we have liftoff. I pause for a second or two to hold my balance. My calves and hamstrings burn as I head for the bathroom. My right knee wobbles and I hear it crunch like balling up newspaper. (Years ago, heading down the steps of an arena for a Stevie Wonder concert, I took a wrong step and the knee went sideways on me. There was no major damage, but I've limped around on it ever since.) My shoulders don't match my stride and the joints pop as I roll them into place. I used to take three Advil every night before bed, so I wouldn't hurt so much in the morning, but I took so many that I was blowing out my capillaries— little red dots started popping up under my skin. So now I gut it out. Have you ever cranked an old car and crossed your fingers that the engine would still fire? Every morning, I feel like a '76 Gremlin.

I lumber into the bathroom. Some days, during that morning pee, I think about something a urologist told me: For every thirty-five pounds you lose, your penis effectively grows by an inch. The fat recedes, you see, revealing what was there all along. If I drop 250 pounds, I might walk around with my fly open all day.

For now, though, I need to get dressed. I put on a T-shirt, step into boxer briefs and jeans. It's hard to put on my pants without tipping over because I'm so top-heavy. So I brace one hand on the dresser for balance. I sit back on the bed to put on my socks because I can't reach down far enough to put them on standing. If I'm wearing lace-up shoes, I have to put them on while I'm on the bed and slide my pants over them. Around the house, it's always slip-ons. God bless Crocs.

The dog pushes through the door—he's got to pee, too—and I follow him out. There are two small steps down from the porch to the sidewalk. I take those two steps carefully. I worry about falling. More to the point, I worry about getting up. Getting off the ground is even more involved than getting out of bed. Every time there's water on the ground—snow or ice or rain—I walk with little penguin steps. Slick mud scares the hell out of me. It's so easy for fat people to fall. We are built out of balance with the world.

I wrote that last sentence wrong. I *made* my body out of balance with the world. I was given a decent frame to start with, but I've done almost nothing to keep it maintained. Of course it's collapsing around me. I've been a shitty homeowner.

We all have those Robert Frost moments where we wonder if the other road would have made all the difference. This is the one I think about the most:

It's the last day of my junior year in high school. I'm walking to class and pass the football coach's office. We've never talked, I don't think. I'm sure he has noticed that I'm the biggest kid in school.

He leans out and congratulates me on my graduation.

Uh, coach, I say, *I'm not graduating. I've got another year.*

He tilts his head and looks at me.

Man, he says. *I wish I'd have known that. We could've made you into a football player.*

I wave and keep walking. His words don't register for a few seconds. Then I start to think about it. Spring practice is over, but the whole summer is ahead. Maybe I should go back and ask him if there's still time.

There's an alternate universe where I turn around and sign up for the team. In that universe I would've lifted weights for the first time in my life. I would've run sprints every day. Even playing the line, where extra bulk is useful, I would've been in the best shape of my life. Maybe I'd be paying the price now: hobbling on torn-up knees, brain-bruised from concussions. There's no way to know how my life would have been different. There's only one thing for sure: When I was given the gift of a chance to exercise hard and get in shape, I turned it down.

That's a decision I've made over and over. There are a million alternate versions of me, stronger and slimmer, wandering out there in the invisible universe, splitting off from me every time I stay on the couch. If they could all get together (I'm not sure this could happen—I haven't seen enough *Star Trek* episodes), I'm guessing they'd look at this version of me and shake their (my) heads, saying the same thing: *Dumbass.*

I know it's what I say to myself.

For a good part of my life I was reasonably athletic. I played baseball and softball in rec leagues and church leagues, usually stationed at first base, where speed is not a requirement. In high school, a group of us played tennis three or four times a week on old asphalt courts where every loose ball rolled toward the same corner. But the sport I loved the most was basketball. When I was twelve, we moved to a house with a park across the road. It had a court with two tilted rims and chain-link nets. I'd run over there after school and shoot by myself, playing the NBA finals in my head, making the game-winning jumper every time, always getting fouled if I missed. Most days, other guys would show up—high school studs, potheads, construction workers still in their boots. Play by ones to fifteen, make 'em take 'em, winners stay on the court, all of us shellacked with sweat, clouds of gnats hovering around our heads like Afros. The game wouldn't stop until somebody caught a pass in the face because it was too dark to see the ball.

Got to stick the big boy, somebody would say. *He can shoot.*

As I got older and bigger, my body couldn't hold up. I sprained my ankles—mostly my right ankle—eight or ten times. If I took a sharp turn when I ran down the court, or came down wrong when I jumped, my ankle crumpled under my weight. All that force coming down on that little tunnel of bone. I fell so many times, and so hard, that I developed a gag reflex: Any time somebody talks about spraining an ankle or breaking a wrist, there's a flash of a second where I want to throw up.

Sometimes I'd get up and keep playing because it didn't really hurt until I stopped. One time in college I went to the infirmary after one of my sprains wasn't healing as fast as it should. The doctor took an X-ray of my right ankle and said the crack from before had healed nicely. I didn't know I had cracked it before. To this day, when I'm not wearing shoes, my ankle clicks every time I take a step.

Slowly, I started giving up sports. Softball first—I played only once or twice after college. Tennis fell away next, sometime around thirty. I quit playing golf when a groundskeeper yelled at me for driving my cart off the path—I didn't want to walk all the way across the fairway to my ball.

I held on to basketball a few more years, had a couple of glory days in pickup games at the Y. But my ankles ached, and my throat surgery had made my windpipe smaller, so it was hard to get enough air. I'd run to one end of the court just in time for the action to go back the other way. The game had lapped me. I quit buying high-tops.

In college, when we played just about every day, this one old guy was always hanging around the campus gym. He wore a Wisconsin tank top—my vague memory is that he had played for the Badgers in the forties or fifties. He couldn't run much, but he had a deadly set shot from the corner. If you got him the ball, it was going up, and it was going in. That's the guy I wanted to be on the back nine of my life. The old guy who could still get it done.

Now when I go to the gym I shoot baskets alone, hoping nobody asks me to get in a game.

Nothing else in my life filled me with instant dread as much as the phrase *shirts vs. skins.*

Every time we split into teams in P.E. class, or in a pickup basketball game, someone would suggest it. It's an easy way to figure out your teammates on the fly. It makes sense if you're a normal boy who looks just fine with his shirt off. I was not a normal boy.

I turned on every bit of charm I had to stay a shirt. I'd look up and smile whenever the shirts' captain was picking. I'd look away whenever the skins chose. It never worked. I always ended up on the skins. I figured this was God's punishment for what I had done to the body he had created.

I'd wait until the last second to peel off my T-shirt. But once it was off, the worst of me was there for everyone to see: my rolls of fat, my breasts sagging down on top of my belly. Most of the time nobody said anything. But I could see their eyes, looking at me and then glancing at their buddies: *Holy shit, look at him!* The one thing about sports, when I was young, was that it gave me a chance to forget I was fat. With my shirt off, I couldn't forget. When I was a skin I couldn't play for shit.

One day in sixth grade they made us play some idiotic game called crab soccer—indoor soccer, but we scuttled around upside down on all fours. I was belly-up and shirtless for everyone to see. Mike, the champion shit-stirrer in our class, scooted over and said: "That boy over there says you got nice tits!"

"WELL HE CAN COME SUCK 'EM THEN!" I yelled to Mike and everybody else, way too loud, failing in my attempt to be a badass fat crab.

One time, playing tennis with my friend Virgil, a girl I liked showed up. In the middle of the match, for reasons I still can't explain—maybe it was sunstroke—I decided to take off my shirt. Incredibly, my running around the tennis court topless did not lead to a date. Years later I found out she had started to date women. I know things don't really work this way, but I still wonder, from time to time, if seeing me flounce around with no shirt on was the thing that flipped her.

Sometimes I'd run into a guy who couldn't leave my chest alone. In high school, at a summer honors program, one guy pinched my nipples so many times I had to threaten to knock him out in front of his friends. A couple years later, in a college flag-football game, a guy reached across the line and squeezed just before the snap. I ran him over on the way to the quarterback. I went back to my spot, burning with murder inside. He switched to the other side of the line.

Here are the two things I know about exercise:

1. Exercise makes you feel better, sleep better, and live longer; it improves your sex life, increases your alertness at work, helps you in almost every way.
2. Exercise doesn't make all that much difference in losing weight.

The reason is one simple equation: To burn off the calories (250) in a single Snickers bar, the average person would have to walk two and a half miles.

This is how I know God has a sick sense of humor. After a night at the Cheesecake Factory, you'd have to cross the country like Forrest Gump.

It doesn't matter what they say on the workout videos and NordicTrack commercials. It doesn't matter how hard you hit the rowing machine or sling the kettlebells. You might end up with great huge muscles under the fat. But multiple medical studies, with a wide range of methods, have shown that diet is far and away the most important factor in weight loss. One 2011 study from the *New England Journal of Medicine* showed that test subjects who went on a diet and exercise program had better health scores than subjects who only dieted . . . but the ones who only dieted lost more weight. Exercise makes you less likely to die of heart disease and diabetes. It builds muscles and eases joint pain. It makes your life better. But all the gym equipment in the world won't make a fat person thin. Anybody who tells you otherwise is trying to sell you something.

This debate always makes me think of Charles Barkley, the NBA Hall of Famer. At six-four (short for a power forward), he weighed around three hundred pounds when he entered the league. His nickname was the Round Mound of Rebound. But somehow he still threw down dunks and outran skinny point guards. It was like watching a bumblebee fly. He was spectacular even with a spare tire. But he didn't turn into a superstar until a few years into his career, when he cut out the postgame pizzas and lost fifty pounds. There's a story about Barkley, as a veteran, telling an overweight teammate: "You could be a great player if you learned just two words: *I'm full.*"

I have never been good with those two words.

And as my body started to break down, anything physical started to feel like a chore. I have always hated chores. When I was a kid, I'd sleep in on days I was supposed to cut the grass. Mama would quit trying to wake me up and just run the lawn mower outside my window until I grumped out of bed. We had an acre of garden where something always needed to be plowed or hoed or picked. We split firewood for our woodstove and built a carport out of railroad ties. Daddy and Mama did most of the work. I bitched and griped and sulked. My folks tried to teach me so much and I refused to learn. I wanted to run and push and sweat but I didn't want it to be work.

The same thing happened when Alix and I bought our first house, a few months after we got married. The place felt like a dream—five and a half acres with a pond and a big garden plot. We talked about working in the yard together and tending to our house as we tended to our new marriage. And that's what we did, especially at first. I'll never forget the day I went out before work and picked 111 tomatoes from our garden, then came back home to find Alix chopping and canning and freezing, the kitchen smeared with red like the climax of a slasher flick. We had fresh vegetables every summer, a field for the dog to run in, hundreds of daylilies lining our driveway.

But then we ended up on opposite work schedules. Each of us had to do chores alone. Pretty soon none of it felt like fun to me. I let things slide and Alix got mad trying to pick up my slack. The house went from something we took joy in to the main thing we argued about. So we sold it. I still drive by there now and then, imagining what we might have done with it if I had made the effort.

This, I've come to believe, is the central complication of my life. I want to do great things, but I don't want any of it to feel like work.

I've earned a paycheck of one kind or another since I was twelve. It's satisfying to do a good job, and on the days my writing goes well, it feels like flying. But I've never gloried in work like a lot of other people do. It's never felt like my purpose. If I won the lottery—forget the Powerball, just a few million bucks—I'd find a beach somewhere and be happy to spend my life watching the tide come in.

On that fantasy beach, my shirt is off, and I look good.

Every body perseveres in its state of rest . . . unless it is compelled to change. Newton's first law is also known as the law of inertia. It is the one law I have followed with devotion. It has kept me on the couch when I needed to get up and move. It has drawn me down the lazy river of life, through too many days where nothing much happens. The law of inertia is seductive as hell.

The law is meant to describe the physical world. But inertia works just as hard on my mind. My willpower has been an object at rest longer than anything else. It is my weakest muscle. I have come to believe, through my own experience and through studying other people for a living, that making a fundamental change of any kind is the hardest thing an adult human being can do.

A couple of years ago, for our fifteenth anniversary, Alix and I decided to go to Europe. We wanted to visit our friend Rosita Boland in Dublin. We wanted to play tourist in London, a place I'd never been. We wanted to see mystery ruins such as Stonehenge. And as we browsed the guidebooks, Alix added another thing to our list: Hadrian's Wall.

In AD 122 the Roman emperor Hadrian built the wall across the narrowest part—seventy-three miles wide—of what is now northern England. It marked the northern border of the Roman Empire. The idea was to keep the "barbarians" in Scotland from getting in. Parts of the wall still survive nearly 1,900 years later. There are hiking trails all around, and several places where you can walk on the wall itself, after you climb the hills to get there.

Hills.

Dammit.

I grew up a flatlander on the Georgia coast. My feeling has always been that hills are pretty when you look at them from the window of a car. Walking up even a slight incline gets me breathing hard right away. I feel like Sisyphus, but I'm the guy and the rock at the same time.

We wanted to see Hadrian's Wall, though. So I had to get ready.

Our neighborhood is mostly flat, but two blocks from our house there's a hill on a side street. It wouldn't challenge even a weekend runner, but on my occasional walks through the neighborhood, I had always avoided it. No more. A couple months before our trip, I walked to the base of the hill, took a couple of deep breaths, and started up.

And stopped about a quarter of the way.

And again about halfway.

And again after that.

A woman blew by me in the street, pushing her baby in a stroller.

The whole loop back to the house took about a mile, and by the end I was washed down in sweat. But I went back the next day, and the one after that, and the one after that. Before long I could tackle the hill with just three stops, then two, then one.

We flew to London, drove out to Stonehenge, spent time with Rosita in Ireland, walked miles every day. I slept like a brick every night. Finally we took a ferry from Dublin to Wales, and a train from there up to northern England. A bus put us out at the Hadrian's Wall visitors' center. It was at the bottom of a hill. The hill looked a lot smaller in the photos.

The path to the wall went up through an active pasture—we had to negotiate sheep, plus what sheep leave behind. That was OK with me. I was looking straight down so I wouldn't have to see how far I had to go. In a couple places, rocks big enough to sit on lay by the side of the path. I wondered if they'd been put there for fat Romans. We stopped and sat until I could catch my breath. Then we pushed on, and a little while later I looked up, surprised to find we were at the top.

The view was worth the trip. To the north, the hill dropped off sharply—no Scots getting up here—and it leveled out into a fantastic field of grass, like God's driving range. Behind us, the sheep looked like toys way down in the pasture. I had to catch my breath again, not because of the journey, but the destination. We stood on the wall someone had built nineteen centuries before, looking down from the top of the hill we had conquered. Alix kissed me. "I'm proud of you," she said.

I was proud, too. Proud and tired and satisfied. A body at rest tends to stay at rest. God knows, my body wants to. But it doesn't *have* to. On top of that ancient wall I could feel it. I still have time to break Newton's law.

MAY

Once you turn fifty, two things happen: AARP starts recruiting you harder than Alabama recruits an all-state linebacker, and your doctor tells you to get a colonoscopy. I sign up for the colonoscopy. It can't be as much of a pain in the ass as the AARP.

To get ready for the colonoscopy, I have to go on a fast and start drinking this stuff called MoviPrep, which tastes like knockoff Gatorade mixed with salt water. I choke down a liter the night before the colonoscopy, and another liter the morning of. It does its awful work. There's nothing left inside my digestive system but air and regret. By the time we get to the clinic, I haven't eaten for thirty-three hours. It's a perfect Starting Over Moment. All the junk in my system has literally been cleaned out. After the colonoscopy I can start filling myself with healthy food, and less of it.

The clinic is running an hour and a half behind. They finally call me back to a little room where I undress and put on one of those fashionable hospital gowns. They hook up an IV and wheel me out on a gurney. We're in the middle of the hallway when the anesthesiologist stops us. By now, I know that anesthesiologists look at fat guys the way families look at the drunk uncle who shows up at the reunion.

"Mr. Tomlinson," he says, looking down at me. "How much do you weigh, again?"

"Around four fifty." Having to say it right in the middle of the nurses and the other patients and everyone.

"Hmm. Let me go talk to the doctor a second."

They wheel me back to the room. A few minutes later, he returns. He says that because of my size, and the throat surgery twenty-two years ago, there's a possibility I'll need a breathing tube. The clinic doesn't have the equipment. So they can't do the colonoscopy here. They'll make a call so I can go straight to the hospital a couple miles away. "You'll thank me for this later," the anesthesiologist says. I'm damn sure not thanking him now.

Now everything goes backward. They take the IV out, I get dressed again, they cut off my little plastic bracelet, Alix walks me to the car. I get almost all the way there before I cry. Waves of self-hate rise up like nausea. It's a colonoscopy clinic. This is what they do. They do thousands a year. And I was too fat for them. Having me there was too big a risk.

It's that feeling I can never shake, of being in the way, of being too much trouble.

The staff at the hospital is kind. They're playing classic rock in the room where they do the procedure—the Stones' "Rock and a Hard Place," which is not the ideal song to hear before a doctor sends a probe up your butt. But they knock me out and I wake up half an hour later, gassy but feeling fine. They find a couple of small polyps, nothing alarming, and tell me to come back in three years.

By the time we leave it has been thirty-nine hours since I've eaten, not that I'm watching the clock. I am most definitely watching the clock. We go to a Mexican place we like. Alix and I often talk about how ordinary food can taste amazing depending on the moment. One year we went to the beach for our anniversary, and after a long walk on the beach we made ham sandwiches with corn chips back at the rental house. They were the best ham sandwiches and corn chips we'd ever had. I say all that to give you the context when I say that burrito at the Mexican place was the best burrito of my life.

But after that, I wasn't that hungry. Most of the time, being embarrassed about my weight pushes me toward food—I eat to numb the pain. This time, something pushes me away. I eat pretty healthy for the rest of the month—enough to feel a difference in the way I move. Maybe the physical cleansing cleaned out something in my brain, too. If so, thank you for your service, MoviPrep. I hope to God we never meet again.

Weight on April 30: 454

Weight on May 31: 449

For the month: -5

For the year: -11

Six

THE AMERICAN WEIGH

My friend and former boss, Frank Barrows, brought up this idea over coffee one day: To understand what dieting is like in America, get a big stack of copies of *O, The Oprah Magazine*—and thumb through the covers like a flipbook.

You can do it online with a Google image search. There's Oprah Winfrey herself, smiling out from every cover, her body an accordion—bigger and smaller and bigger again—as the months and years go by. Read the headlines and it sounds like a debate the two Oprahs are having with each other:

What's Holding You Back?

Celebrate Who You Are Now!

Fresh Start!

Life Is a Banquet!

Are You Ready for a Change?

Let It Go!

Oprah is a billionaire with the resources to pay for the freshest food, the smartest nutritionists, the most skilled personal trainers. She famously dragged a red wagon full of fat onto the stage of her show after losing sixty-seven pounds on a liquid protein diet. Another time, she ran the Marine Corps Marathon. Over and over, she loses weight. Over and over, it finds her again. Her brains and charm made her a success. Those extra pounds make her the most beloved celebrity in America. As high as she flies, her weight pulls her down to the rest of us.

If Oprah beat her weight problem once and for all, we might not need Oprah anymore. We cheer for her when she's winning, we root for her when she's losing, and she gets paid either way. But I wonder how much she would give to be exactly the size she wants to be. I wonder how many billions it would be worth to her never to worry about her weight again.

It would be worth almost anything to me.

The first diet plan I remember was pills. Mama took me to a diet doctor when I was eleven or twelve and already growing out of the husky sizes at Sears. I don't remember him saying anything about eating right or exercise. I just remember a long cabinet full of white plastic bottles. At the end of the visit he gave me a handful of pills that looked as bright and happy as Skittles. Looking back, I'm pretty sure at least some were amphetamines. They didn't curb my appetite—I was still sneaking into the fridge at night for bologna sandwiches or banana pudding. But the next day I could run up and down the basketball court for hours. This seemed to me to be a good trade-off.

The next diet plan I remember was candy. They were these little chocolates that came in a box like a Whitman's sampler. They were called Ayds, which turned out years later to be an extremely unfortunate name. They were supposed to have some sort of appetite suppressant. They did not suppress my appetite enough to keep me from eating five or six instead of one.

I remember the *first* time carbohydrates were bad for you, back in the seventies. The lunch counter at Woolworth's in Brunswick sold a diet plate of a hamburger patty on a lettuce leaf with a side of cottage cheese. My mom and I stared at the picture on the menu like it was a platypus at the zoo. We pretended to care about carbs for a while. Mama even bought a little carbohydrate guide she kept in her pocketbook. It said biscuits and cornbread were bad for us. It didn't stay in her pocketbook long.

I've gone through diets like Gene Simmons through groupies. I've done low-fat and low-carb and low-calorie, high-protein and high-fruit and high-fiber. I've tried the Mediterranean and taken my talents to South Beach. I've shunned processed foods and guzzled enough SlimFast to drown a rhino. I've eaten SnackWell's cookies (low-fat, tons of sugar) and chugged Tab (no sugar, tons of chemicals, faint whiff of kerosene). I've been told, at different times, that eggs, bacon, toast, cereal, and milk are all bad for you. I've also been told that each one of those things is an essential part of a healthy diet. My brain is fogged enough at breakfast. Don't fuck with me like this.

I started to say something like *Name a diet, I've tried it.* But that's not true because somebody invents a new diet every day, and half the time the author gets a *New York Times* best seller out of it. Here's a quick Amazon listing of top-selling diet books:

> *The Negative Calorie Diet: Lose Up to 10 Pounds in 10 Days with 10 All You Can Eat Foods*
> *The Fast Metabolism Diet: Eat More Food and Lose More Weight*
> *10-Day Green Smoothie Cleanse: Lose Up to 15 Pounds in 10 Days!*
> *The Wild Diet: Get Back to Your Roots, Burn Fat, and Drop Up to 20 Pounds in 40 Days*
> *Super Shred: The Big Results Diet: 4 Weeks, 20 Pounds, Lose It Faster!*

These diets are all hugely popular, and they all fail what I call the Carny Test. The Carny Test applies whenever somebody is trying to sell you something: If you can imagine a guy in a straw hat hollering it outside a carnival tent, it's probably a bad deal. "Step right up! Lose up to 10 pounds in 10 days with 10 all-you-can-eat foods!" You would never spend a ticket on that at the county fair. But people pay thirty bucks a pop for the books, and most of the time, the only thing that gets smaller is their bank balance.

Here are the two things I have come to believe about diets:

1. Almost any diet works in the short term.
2. Almost no diets work in the long term.

A diet works in the short term because it's better than no diet at all. If you ate nothing but deep-dish pizza for the next month—pause with me a second to daydream about eating deep-dish pizza for a month—as long as you didn't OVEReat deep-dish pizza, you'd probably lose weight. You'd take in fewer calories just by limiting your portions and paying attention. (I do not endorse the Deep-Dish Diet, and neither does your lower GI tract.)

But even a diet that's working grinds you down over time. If I go low-carb or no-carb for a while, I start to drop some pounds. I also get that little fizz of energy that comes from being morally superior. *No, YOU take the bread. I'll nourish myself with WILLPOWER.* But at some point I notice that every street in town has a bakery on it, and sometimes for lunch it would be nice to have a sandwich, and I go to a party and there's a bowl of hummus and hummus is (kind of) good for you, but I can't just scoop it with my finger—oh look, there's some pita chips . . .

Oprah invested forty million dollars in Weight Watchers not long ago. I've spent maybe four hundred dollars on Weight Watchers over the years. Based on our respective net worths, that seems about right. Weight Watchers is the closest plan to what I'm trying to do with my Three-Step Diet. It's based on counting calories (WW converts calories into points to make counting easier) and it's intended for slow, steady weight loss. You can even do Weight Watchers online now, which makes sense, because the problem with Weight Watchers is the meetings. They always felt strange and awkward to me, even when I was among friends. The Weight Watchers rep is always a little too cheery. The members generally sit there in silence except for the occasional mumbled confessional. It's like a corporate team-building seminar for overweight people. Most people are just there to do the weigh-in. We'd all empty our pockets and take off our belts and shoes, as if we were going through airport security, just to shave off a pound or two on the scale. I always hoped somebody would go the full Ultimate Fighting weigh-in route and strip down to their underwear, then stand around and talk shit to everybody who didn't lose as much weight. Maybe there would be a pull-apart brawl. My mind wandered a lot at Weight Watchers meetings.

It's also possible that Weight Watchers pissed me off because they never had a scale big enough for me. (How do you know you're *really* fat? When you're too fat for the Weight Watchers scale.)

I don't know if my simple Three-Step Diet will work. Some days it feels like capitalism—the worst system ever invented, except for all the others. Mostly, though, it feels like baseball. Mood swings don't work in baseball. It's too long a season. So you have to enjoy the wins, but not too much, and worry over the losses, but not too much.

Some days I overeat. Other days I don't walk enough. Some days I fly off the rails and end up facedown in a pizza. My Fitbit log swings back and forth like the Flying Dutchman at the state fair. One day I ate 1,603 calories and burned 3,343—more than half a pound to the good. The very next day I burned 4,205—but ate 4,917. That's nearly double the recommended intake. It was a long travel day. I had a one-night stand with a double cheeseburger and a chocolate shake.

But I'm winning more than I'm losing. And I'm not day-trading my own body by switching to the diet of the month. By losing weight this way, I know it'll go more slowly. I'll never experience the joy of having somebody's jaw drop because I'm six sizes smaller than I was the last time they saw me. But I hope I won't have the pain of backsliding all the way to where I started.

A diet is no good if it works for just a week or ten days or a month. It has to be something you can live with (apologies to Shakespeare) tomorrow, and tomorrow.

And tomorrow.

The most depressing five-word Google search I can think of—and I can think of a LOT of depressing five-word Google searches—is "gained all the weight back." Not long ago I read a beautiful piece by a writer who lost 125 pounds in a year. He linked to a story that had inspired him by another writer who lost 153 pounds in a year. When I clicked through to the second writer's story, I landed on his website. His recent tweets ran down the side of the page. One of them said how proud he was to have been an inspiration . . . even though he had gained most of the weight back. Losing weight is not the hard part. The hard part is living with a diet for years, maybe the rest of your life. That's why almost no diets work in the long run.

When we go on a diet—especially a crash diet—our own bodies turn against us. Nutritional studies have shown that hunger-suppressing hormones in our bodies dwindle when we lose weight. Other hormones—the ones that warn us we need to eat—tend to rise. Our bodies beg us to gorge at the first sign of deprivation. This makes sense when you think about the history of humankind. There were no Neanderthal foodies. They ate to survive. They went hungry for long stretches. Their bodies sent up alarms telling them they'd better find something to eat. Our DNA still harbors that fear that we'll starve. This wasn't a problem when there was a chance we really might waste away. But now most of us have access to food that is more abundant, cheaper, and more addictive than at any other time in human history. Our bodies haven't caught up to the modern world. Our cells think we're storing up fat for a hard winter when actually it's just happy hour at Chili's.

Even worse, when people succeed at losing a lot of weight, their bodies slam on the brakes of their metabolism. Scientists from the National Institutes of Health found this out most recently by studying contestants from the eighth season of *The Biggest Loser*. The *New York Times* did a big story on the study. It showed a photo of one of the contestants, Sean Algaier, and said he was now a pastor at a church in Charlotte. The church is a fifteen-minute drive from my house.

A few days later, I went out there to meet Sean. His office has sturdy chairs.

. . .

At the time we talk, Sean is thirty-six years old, a husband and a father of three. He is funny and open and says *dude* a lot. He keeps his zero-calorie sports drinks cold in his son's Transformers lunchbox.

In 2009, when they were living in Tulsa, his wife found out about a *Biggest Loser* casting call in Oklahoma City. She told Sean he was going. He went thinking he had no chance—something like 350,000 people around the country tried out for the show. Even when he made it to the final screening group of forty—they all met in Los Angeles to see how everyone got along—he thought everybody else was more interesting. But back home, with NBC's cameras watching, he got the phone call that he was in.

He lasted on the show just three weeks, mostly by his choice. In that time he lost thirty-six pounds—dropping from 444 to 408—and volunteered to be kicked off because others on his team were struggling, and he thought they needed the trainers and counselors more than he did. He believed he could keep losing weight at home. And he did. He got all the way down to 289—a total of 155 pounds. He celebrated by running a marathon in Tulsa. It took him almost seven hours, but he crossed the finish line. "You get to a place where nothing will stop you from doing whatever it is that you want to do," he says.

But he did stop. And then he slid backward.

The day we talk, about seven years after *The Biggest Loser*, Sean had recently been in the hospital briefly for cellulitis—a bacterial rash on his legs. His doctor told him he had type 2 diabetes. Sean went back home, dieted hard, and lost twenty pounds in a week and a half. He had weighed in the day before we spoke. He was at 444. Exactly where he'd been when he started on the show.

No one thing tipped him. His job in Tulsa wasn't going the way he had hoped, so he and his family packed up and moved. He had the normal stress of any parent raising three young children. He spent time in counseling and it opened some old wounds—he had been in foster care for a few years when he was small, then had hard times with an adoptive family. It all rolled up on him.

"I developed this pattern of feeling worthless," he says. "And so, I guess in my darkest places now, there is still a little bit of a feeling of worthlessness."

Like me—like so many people—he tamped down those feelings with food. He'd go to a Charlotte breakfast joint called the Flying Biscuit and gorge on biscuits and gravy. He'd dig into the stashes of cake and doughnuts they kept around for the kids. On his best days he could avoid those things, or just have a bite or two. But when he felt down, he dove in with both hands.

He knows he can lose a lot of weight. He's done it. But when the scientists studied him and the other contestants—before the show, afterward, and six years later—they made a heartbreaking discovery.

Other studies had already shown that the body's metabolism slows down as people lose weight, which means they have to eat fewer and fewer calories to keep losing. But this study showed that, for the contestants who lost weight quickly, their metabolism kept slowing *even when they started gaining weight again*. Basically, however fat they had been, that's what their bodies wanted them to be.

Sean remembers all the tests the researchers ran—blood work, sleep studies, assessments in an egg-shaped thing called the Bod Pod to get a precise measurement of body fat. He had lost touch with some of his fellow contestants and didn't realize that many of them had gained their weight back, too. He agreed to talk to the *Times* for their story, but when it came out it was an anvil on his chest. He had given speeches around the country telling people they could lose weight the way he had. He felt like a hypocrite: "It's like, anyone that had inspiration from me before . . . now I'm disqualified from being inspirational."

The response to the story surprised him. People were encouraged that he was still trying. They supported him no matter what. The people who loved him still loved him. Sean and I talk about this for a while. We struggle with the same fears. A lot of the time, because we haven't loved ourselves, we don't think other people will love us. We don't think we deserve to be loved. We both turn to food for a moment of peace.

"I'd look in the mirror, and I'm like, what is wrong with me?" Sean says. "Why can't I feel fulfilled or happy? And for me, the feeling was like, if my stomach was full, then I was comfortable. I've eaten; I'm good; I'm full."

He looks at me across his desk. I nod back. I know exactly what he means.

We're about the same size right now, Sean and I. We are two fat men trying hard to be something else. He found a better version of himself and lost it again. I've never seen my better version.

Sean has nothing but good things to say about his time on *The*

Biggest Loser. I believe him, but I can't stand the show. I hate the way they run the contestants until it looks like they're about to die. I hate the double-meaning dagger of the title. I hate, more than anything, the way they make the men take their shirts off when they weigh in, all their shame displayed for ratings' sake, so viewers will stare in disgust and tune in again next week. Under all the inspiration is the rancid smell of a freak show. And I hate it so much because I know it would probably work. If I had to take my shirt off over and over on national TV, I would goddamn sure lose weight. Or die trying.

But no one lives on camera forever. What happens when the lights go off, and the support staff goes home, and our own bodies work against us?

Sean is a pastor, and I am a believer, and so we talk about God for a while. I tell Sean that when it comes to my weight, sometimes it feels as if I'm set up to fail. Sean sees it differently: "I think God is like, *Look, son, I really need you to listen to me.*"

What causes us to fail: the devil's whisper in our ears, or the angel we ignore? At some point it doesn't matter. The number on the scale reads the same.

Eat less and exercise.

That's what some of you are saying right now. That's what some of you have said the whole time you've been reading this book. That's what some of you say—maybe not out loud, but you say it—every time you see a fat person downing fried eggs in a diner, or overstuffing a bathing suit on the beach, or staring out from one of those good-Lord-what-happened-to-her? stories in the gossip magazines.

Eat less and exercise.

Yes sir, yes ma'am, thank you for the advice. We will take that under consideration—me, and Sean, and Oprah, and all the millions of others like us. Eat less and exercise. Such a simple thing.

What I want you to understand, more than anything else, is that telling a fat person *Eat less and exercise* is like telling a boxer *Don't get hit.*

You act as if there's not an opponent.

Losing weight is a fucking rock fight. The enemies come from all sides. The deluge of marketing telling us to eat worse and eat more. The culture that has turned food into one of the last acceptable vices. Our families and friends who want us to share in their pleasure. Our own body chemistry, dragging us back to the table out of fear that we'll starve.

On top of all that, some of us fight holes in our souls that a boxcar of doughnuts couldn't fill.

My compulsion to eat comes from all those places. I'm almost never hungry in the physical sense. But I'm always craving an emotional high, the kind that comes from making love, or being in the crowd for great live music, or watching the sun come up over the ocean. And I'm always wanting something to counter the low, when I'm anxious about work or arguing with family or depressed for reasons I can't understand.

There's a scene in the movie *Monster's Ball* that I think about a lot. Halle Berry's character, Leticia, has lost almost everything. Her husband went to the electric chair. Her son was hit by a car and died. She winds up in her living room with Hank, Billy Bob Thornton's character, who has been through some shit of his own. They barely know each other but they start to talk, and she starts to cry, and then she turns to him and starts taking off her clothes. "Can you make me feel good?" she begs him, and her voice goes low and ragged. "Just make me feel good."

That's all I want sometimes. Just something to make me feel good. At the right time, or in the right place, I can find something higher: satisfaction, contentment, fulfillment. But food brings me the quickest gratification, the swiftest bliss. Those feelings aren't the same as the higher ones. But they almost rhyme.

Just make me feel good, my whole being begs. So I rise like a sleepwalker and head for the fridge.

JUNE

The hardest part of South Dakota was the stupid green dinosaur.

A group of us flew up to Rapid City to see our friends Gina Nania and David Gwinn for Gina's sixtieth birthday. We packed as much into three days as we could. We marveled at the Black Hills. We saw Mount Rushmore at night, the presidents' heads hovering in the dark like spooks. We clambered around the Badlands, which look like the Grand Canyon turned inside out. We saw bighorn sheep and herds of buffalo and a billion prairie dogs. We laughed at a wild burro that poked its snout in our car and scratched its chin on the edge of the window. We visited Wall Drug, which was like the entire tourist strip of Myrtle Beach condensed into a bouillon cube.

Alix and I walked miles every day and slept like boards every night. We got closer to some of our favorite people. The whole trip was fantastic.

Except when I looked up from the bottom of the hill at the green concrete dinosaur.

Five dinosaurs, actually. They're part of Dinosaur Park, a tourist attraction in Rapid City since the 1930s. They're all painted green, and you can see the big one—the brontosaurus—from just about anywhere in town. It's an obvious place to visit if you're tooling around Rapid City. We went on the first day. The only thing was, we had to climb up the side of a hill to get there.

I didn't mind climbing a hill to see Hadrian's Wall. I wasn't crazy about climbing a hill to see concrete dinosaurs.

This is what I do when we talk about trying something hard. I grumble about it. I convince myself it's not worth doing anyway. I sigh and mutter and bitch under my breath, knowing Alix will hear me but hoping nobody else does.

Later on I found out there had been a lot of email traffic about me before the trip even started. We were up there during the week of the Crazy Horse Volksmarch, a six-mile hike that's one of the rare chances every year to get a close look at the massive Crazy Horse mountain carving. Our group of friends includes some die-hard hikers, and they hoped everybody would go on the Volksmarch. There was no way I could do six miles, especially if part of the trail was uphill. Notes got passed back and forth. In the end, half the group hiked, the rest of us went to Deadwood, and we met up later on. It all turned out fine. But I suspect everybody would've gone to Crazy Horse if I hadn't been around.

And now, this damn hill. I grumbled and started to climb.

The path didn't have great railings—they were really low in places, and I had to hunch over to hang on. The steps got steeper. I had to stop a couple times. Our friend Chuck Lampe, who could've bounded up the steps two at a time, hung back and talked to me as I caught my breath. I pulled myself up the last few steps to the top, ready to hate the stupid green dinosaurs.

The view was breathtaking.

I'm enough of a flatlander that looking down from the top of anything is still a surprise. The city pooled down below us, and lights from houses twinkled in the hills. A breeze came off the prairie and cooled my sweat. I'm from the coast and Alix grew up on Lake Michigan. We both miss the wind. You don't get much wind in Charlotte. But here it was on the first night of our trip. The rest of the weekend was gravy once we felt that wind.

It turns out this way almost every time something is physically challenging. I don't want to do it. I try to get out of it. I grumble about having to do it. Then I do it and it's great. It seems like I would remember, having repeated the pattern this long. But my rat brain—the part that operates on fear and instinct—always wants to say no. My rat brain cares only about survival. It doesn't know the value of doing something hard. And it has no understanding of why it felt so good to have the wind in my face at the top of the hill.

I need a poster that says DON'T LISTEN TO THE RAT BRAIN. Maybe it could have a green dinosaur on it.

Weight on May 31: 449

Weight on June 30: 444

For the month: -5

For the year: -16

Seven

ACCOMMODATIONS

The first time I flew on a commercial airplane was when I was twenty-three. My friend Perry Beard had won the ticket lottery to the 1987 Final Four in New Orleans. There were lots of firsts on that trip: first visit to the French Quarter, first beignets, first time approached by a hooker. (Hooker: "Buy me a drink?" Me, stammering: "Uh, we were just, uh, leaving.") My friend David Duclos drove out there from Georgia with me, but he had to go home early, so I booked a one-way flight back. The plane was half-empty. The guys from a band called Big Audio Dynamite—you might know them as Mick Jones's offshoot of the Clash—sprawled out behind me, dozing and moaning. If you fly out of New Orleans in the morning, chances are most people on the plane will be hungover.

Nobody else was in my row, so I had room to stretch out. But when I went to buckle my seat belt, the two halves wouldn't reach. I didn't know about seat belt extensions. My panicked (and possibly hungover) twenty-three-year-old brain didn't even know to ask. So

I covered my lap with a blanket. The flight attendant did her pre-flight check and walked right on past—she might have been hung-over, too. So I white-knuckled the takeoff and landing, gripping the armrests like barnacles.

I dreaded getting on a plane again. But the next time, as soon as I sat down, a flight attendant brought me an extension. I looked at it as if all the mysteries of the universe had been explained.

By now I've learned to navigate my life as a fat man. I know what to ask for when I need it. I've figured out escape hatches and work-arounds. But that low note of dread never goes away when I have to make my way through public spaces. Nothing ever quite fits.

Now, when I get on a plane, I catch the flight attendant's eye and make a little seat-belt pantomime. They always know what that means. Sometimes they hand me the extension without looking, as if they're passing me a bag of weed on a street corner. Part of me is grateful that they don't make a fuss. But part of me feels like it really is contraband, like something I'm not supposed to have, because this is a place where I don't belong.

One other quick seat-belt story.

A few years ago I went down to spring training in Florida with my longtime friend Joe Posnanski and three other writers: Chris Jones, Kevin Van Valkenburg, and Michael Schur. We all bonded right away, talking about storytelling and sports, laughing over two-hour breakfasts, watching baseball in the sun. It was one of the best weeks of my life. Except when we had to ride in the car.

Joe had rented an SUV, so he drove. It was clear that I would get the passenger seat and the other three would squeeze into the back. Chris and Mike are normal-sized. Kevin played linebacker at Montana. Those guys got to know one another well.

I felt terrible for them. But the worst part was that my seat belt wouldn't fit around me. I adjusted the seat and sucked in my gut as tight as I could, but the latch stopped an inch from the buckle. When Joe started the car, the warning bell would ring.

Ding. Ding. Ding.

Every couple of miles it tolled again.

Ding. Ding. Ding.

We ignored it, talked over it, but sometimes we were quiet for a minute and—

Ding. Ding. Ding.

—I knew what everybody was thinking.

It took me a whole day to figure out what to do. I slipped the belt behind my back and buckled it. If we wrecked, I'd have a faceful of windshield. But at least the goddamn dinging went away.

Some people pick their cars for the engine, or the color, or the gas mileage, or the stereo. The first thing I check is the seat belt. About half the time, it doesn't fit. And if it doesn't fit, nothing else matters.

As a people, we are getting too big for our britches.

Companies that supply furniture to schools are having to sell big-and-tall desks because kids can't fit into the regular ones anymore.

Ballparks are making their seats bigger. When Notre Dame

recently updated its football stadium—which opened in 1930—it gave up more than three thousand seats by redrawing the boundaries on the benches in the stands. Now the seats are eighteen inches wide instead of sixteen, to make room for wider Fighting Irish butts.

Movie theater seats are even wider—twenty-three inches on average these days, up from twenty inches in 1990. The aisles are deeper, too, and most theaters have armrests you can lift out of the way.

Ambulance companies now build gurneys that can hold up to 1,600 pounds, up from the old standard of 800; they're pulled into the ambulance by a winch. CT scanners have grown from sixty centimeters in diameter to eighty because people were getting stuck inside.

The average width of an American casket used to be twenty-four inches. Now it's twenty-eight, and a company called Goliath Casket makes a coffin fifty-two inches wide that can hold one thousand pounds of flesh and bones. They ship out half a dozen a month.

Poking around on Goliath Casket's website, I found a page with advice for funeral directors. The page is titled "Solving the Problems." A few highlights:

> *The easiest way to handle an obese funeral is to refer the family to your competitor, but that rarely works, especially if you picked up the body strapped to two hospital mattresses (oh—the pain!) . . .*

It goes on from there to tips for moving the body—turns out an engine hoist works well—to double-checking the size and location of the burial plot, just to make sure there's enough room.

You might read that and decide on cremation. Good luck. Many crematoriums can't handle oversized bodies.

Fat people are trouble all the way to the grave.

Not long after Alix and I moved into the house we live in now, we redid our guest bathroom. Our house was built in 1929, and the bathroom had a crack in the floor that turned out to be a symptom of a bigger problem underneath. We had to rip everything out and get a new bathroom built. (It's still the nicest room in our house.) We liked it so much that we started taking showers in there. After a few months, I noticed that water was pooling in one spot in the middle of our new tub. It was the place where I stood when I showered. I had bent the floor of the steel tub.

Of all the places I end up during a normal day, I worry about bathrooms most.

If it's a public restroom, I head straight for the handicapped stall. One of these days I expect to finish my business and open the door to find a pissed-off guy in a wheelchair. But for me, most regular stalls are like trying to squeeze into a Porsche. If I have to sit, I ease down slowly and listen for creaks. One of my greatest fears is sitting on a wall-mounted toilet and having it snap under my weight, dumping me on the floor and soaking me in pee and toilet water.

I have to stand up to wipe. Sitting down, I can't reach.

Over the years I've busted multiple toilet seats. I've worn out the springs on several easy chairs and at least two couches. I mash down my side of the mattress so much that Alix rolls downhill toward me in the night, which works out great for me but is not so fun for her. One time I leaned back too hard in my old Chrysler LeBaron and broke the bucket seat. I jammed a milk crate behind it to prop it up and drove that way for years.

In college, at the apartment of a girl I was trying to impress, I sat in her wooden chair. I could hear it start to crack but I couldn't get out of it fast enough. The whole thing exploded into tindersticks.

NASCAR drivers talk about "driving with your ass." Their cars are slung so close to the ground that their butt muscles can sense how the car is handling the track. I drive with my ass any time I sit in an unfamiliar chair. I'm constantly gauging how it feels under me, if there's any hint of bending or cracking. When a rickety chair is the only choice, I sit as lightly as I can, and I sweat, and I pray. Another recurring fear: A chair will crack into pieces under me, and one of the shards will impale my thigh. I'll die right there on the floor, from blood loss or embarrassment.

My friends know all this instinctively. The other night a group of us went to a coffee shop with mismatched chairs. They left me an armless chair that looked like it was made from butcher block. If we sit at a rectangular table, they'll save me a spot at one end. It's our unspoken contract.

Bottlenecks make me nervous—doorways, turnstiles, anywhere people are trying to crowd from one place to another. I'm not claustrophobic. I just can't shake the feeling that I'm in the way. "*Everybody's* in the way," Alix says, and of course she's right. But I'm always swiveling and shuffling and looking for a way to the edge. I'm useless at crowded parties. My voice doesn't carry to begin with, and I'm constantly worried about clogging the flow of traffic. Most of the time I end up in the corner, inspecting the host's book collection.

Here's one that happens four or five times a year. I'll be in a hotel or office building somewhere and punch the button for the elevator. The doors open, and it's crowded inside—tight but not completely full. I could probably wedge my way in there. But I can always see a couple of people looking at me with dread. Somebody will glance over at the panel. I know what that person is looking for. The load limit.

It doesn't matter if I'm running late, or if I'm tired of traveling and just want to get to my room. I never get on that elevator. I just take a step back and say I'll wait. Somebody always sighs in relief as the doors close.

If I'm going to a concert or a ball game, even a movie, I get there early. Part of it is that I like watching things get set up—baseball players taking batting practice, roadies working on the drum kit. But mostly I want to make sure the seat works.

The first time I went to Fenway Park, on a baseball trip with Perry, I couldn't buy an aisle seat. The game was sold out and we had to buy tickets off the street to get in. Fenway was built in 1912 and most of the seats are the same ones they had back then. Based on the room in the seats, Americans used to be about a third of our current size. Fenway is the best ballpark in American sports, a place I'd always dreamed of going, but I was crammed in like a champagne cork—if I had popped out, I'd have landed on the pitcher's mound. I've been back a few times since then, and have had better seats, but I still get a little shudder when I see all those fans mashed together on TV.

I'm obsessive about knowing where I'm going to sit. When I was music writer for the *Charlotte Observer*, it drove me crazy that I never got to pick where I sat. My seat was whatever the promoters had left once they'd taken care of VIPs, employees, radio contest winners, and so on. It was usually near the front, but almost always in the middle of a row. When Janet Jackson played the Charlotte Coliseum, I was stuffed into a seat directly behind Stephanie Mills, the star of the original Broadway version of *The Wiz*. My legs were sticking out and spread wide because I couldn't fit all the way back into the seat. The back of Stephanie's head rested a couple inches from my crotch. Sometimes I wonder if Stephanie ever goes inside a sweaty gym and the smell reminds her of "Rhythm Nation" for reasons she can't quite place.

Not long ago I was back in the music game for a bit, doing a story for *Our State*—a magazine about North Carolina—on singer Rhiannon Giddens. She was playing in Charlotte at the McGlohon Theater, a beautiful old church converted into a concert hall. This time I had bought a ticket—five rows back on the aisle. But the McGlohon's seats are irregular. It took some wiggling just to get into the seat. Then I got up to talk to some friends. When I came back, just before the show was about to start, a large woman was in the seat next to mine. Both of us would've been miserable.

Slow panic.

I headed for the balcony, climbing a couple flights of steep stairs. When I got to the top I was washed down in sweat. The houselights went down. I slipped into the back of the balcony and asked the usher if there was any open space. He pointed me to a couple of rows in the back, the only unsold seats in the house. I found a place and sat down just as Rhiannon started singing. It was still a good spot—the McGlohon isn't a big theater—and the music was so powerful that, like any great art, it pulled me out of time and space. I took my notes and did my job and only once in a while did I look around and notice that nobody was sitting anywhere near me.

This is where being fat leaves me. Panicked and sweaty. Isolated and alone.

Husky is the first size I remember. It was on the tags of my shirts. I would always cut out the tags, and the little stubs left behind would make my neck itch. It was worth it. The evidence of my huskiness was gone. As if you couldn't just look at me and tell.

It's not hard to remember the clothes I've really loved. It's a short list. My brother, Ronald, gave me an old football practice jersey that I wore for years—until the day in a pickup basketball game that a guy reached for the ball, hooked the jersey instead, and ripped it in half. I had a three-quarter-sleeve Hawaiian Tropic shirt that I wore until it shredded. I had a T-shirt for Penn tennis balls that lasted until the collar came off. I had a green corduroy hat from the Masters that fit just right—hats are hard for me to find because my head is a size eight. It drowned in the river on a fishing trip.

Fat people find clothes in weird places. One time I found a stash of 6X polo shirts at a gas station in Tuscaloosa, Alabama. I didn't really need gas station polo shirts, but I almost bought a couple because who knows when I'll find one next? In small towns overweight people might have to go to the army navy store or the discount outlet, where they mash a rack of pants in between used car parts and last year's toys. The year we were in Boston, the best big-and-tall shop was in the basement of an old shut-down public library. I don't buy clothes online unless I'm ninety-nine percent sure they're going to fit, because most things don't. I'm one of five American white guys over fifty who don't own a pair of Dockers. They don't fit my thighs. If they did I'd be fine with wearing Dockers every day, even if it meant a sudden urge to listen to Huey Lewis and the News again.

Many guys like me shop at what is now known as Destination XL—I'll always call it by its old name, Casual Male. In many cities it's the only place for men to find big-and-tall clothes. Up until a few years ago, Casual Male's shirts topped out at 6X and pants topped out at size sixty. Those are my sizes. There are other guys in Charlotte who must be the same size, because sometimes every 6X shirt will be gone. I've learned to call ahead. I used to worry that if I kept getting fatter, I'd never be able to buy clothes in a store again. But Casual Male's sizes have gone up. You can routinely find 7X or 8X shirts, or pants up to sixty-eight or seventy. People who wear those sizes probably weigh more than five hundred pounds. Now there are enough people like that to put those clothes on the rack. The place I went to in Boston—it's called the Big Men's Stout Men's Shop—carried waist sizes up to eighty-eight, and shirts up to 12X. Basically, clothes for people who can no longer leave the house.

Casual Male makes good stuff, the prices are reasonable, and the salespeople help but don't hover. The doors of the dressing rooms have little chalkboards on the outside, and the clerks mark the occupied rooms with sly affirmations: SUPERSTAR or BOSS or PLAYA. Sometimes I'll take half a dozen shirts and three or four pairs of pants in there. Sometimes nothing fits. I can count on one good meltdown a year in the Casual Male dressing room.

A few years ago Casual Male expanded from clothes and added a division called Living XL. Now you can buy a bicycle made with reinforced steel and an extra-wide seat. Or if you're a little less active, a camp chair that holds up to a thousand pounds. Or if you're less active still, a recliner that tips forward to help you get out.

Scrolling through the catalog is a glimpse into a nightmare future: *Yep, I could use that . . . nope, don't need that yet . . . God, I hope I never need that.*

In a way, I'm glad this stuff exists. It used to be impossible for fat people to find something as simple as a comfortable chair. Now, if you have the money, you can outfit your whole house. Right now I'm writing this from a supersized office chair that probably did not exist twenty years ago.

The problem is not that all this stuff exists. The problem is that it needs to. Destination XL is a destination where no one wants to go. But millions of us are walking that way, stopping every so often to rest.

Overweight people are now a solid majority in America. So it makes sense that there's an increasing movement to defend fatness, and even celebrate it.

The National Association to Advance Fat Acceptance (which has been around since the sixties) fights "to eliminate discrimination based on body size." Fat-positive advocates demand more selection in stores and more people who look like them in magazine ads and on TV. The attention has worked. Dove, the beauty-product brand, has curvy regular women (not models or actresses) in its ads. *Sports Illustrated* featured the gorgeous plus-sized model Ashley Graham in its swimsuit issue. All this gets filtered back through the columnists and bloggers and YouTubers who tell their own stories of dealing with being overweight, struggling with how the world sees them, and finding joy and peace in their own bodies.

Part of this is common sense. Overweight doesn't always equal unhealthy. Some people carry extra pounds naturally.

Part of it is anger. A lot of fat people feel they don't get the jobs and promotions they deserve, and studies tend to back them up. Fat people are tired of being made fun of. There aren't many jokes you can tell in our sensitive society without getting in some kind of trouble, but fat jokes are always safe. My stance on fat jokes is the same as my stance on every other kind of joke: Nothing's out of bounds. Humor is risk. Just make a little effort. Most fat jokes are lazy. A political writer I admire—one of the best in the world, smart and insightful—can't help himself when he mentions Chris Christie. He goes for the fat joke every time. It's like waving a ribbon in front of a cat.

So I understand the impulse to stick a flag in Plus Size Nation and tell everybody else to fuck off. It's my own impulse sometimes. I'm thrilled for people who are happy and healthy and content with their size. I admire writers such as Lindy West, who in her work (especially her amazing book *Shrill*) makes the body-positive case with such logic and force that it's hard to argue otherwise.

So I'm not going to argue. I'm just going to speak for myself.

I don't want the world to expand to make room for me. It's not good for me, and it's not good for the world. I need to make myself fit. That's not conforming to some outdated notion of what the human body should look like, or aiming for some unattainable standard. It's just trying to walk through the world without a headwind. It's being not so goddamn worried about going to every new place or trying any new thing.

All of us, I think, have this disconnect between the face we put out to the world and the one we wear alone. I try my best to hide my fears at all the ways the world doesn't fit me. It doesn't always work, and even when it does, I'm constantly looking around for the next thing I might break, the next place I'm too big to squeeze through. Maybe I should just elbow my way through the tight spaces, mold the world to my shape. That feels liberating. It also feels like giving myself permission to live the life that's destroying me. The world doesn't fit me because I'm not supposed to be this big. Maybe other people are. Not me.

That word *husky* has stuck with me since I was a kid. It makes me think of a literal husk, something that's supposed to be let go when the time is right. My husk has hung on way too long. For me to find peace, I have to shed it.

JULY

Alix and I spend our anniversary in Greenville, South Carolina, one of the most underrated towns in America. It's just a two-hour drive from Charlotte, but we'd never hung out there. The one and only thing we've regretted about getting married is that we picked the wrong month. Everywhere we've been for our anniversary has been brutally hot. We should have gone with October, but we got married in a fever. We went with July. And in Greenville it's ninety-six degrees.

Still, we walk all day. We walk up the street to the Saturday morning farmers' market for breakfast. We walk down to Falls Park, where a wide and beautiful waterfall runs right through the middle of town. We walk over the falls on the Liberty Bridge. We walk to the ballpark where the Greenville Drive minor league team plays. No game that day, but the park is gorgeous. Shoeless Joe Jackson's old house is right across the street.

This is the way we'd always pictured our life together. We love strolling through downtowns, poking around in galleries and bookstores, people-watching. Sometimes we curl up on the couch together and daydream about the places we want to go, the things we've never seen, or haven't seen together. Machu Picchu. Greece and Rome. Yosemite and Yellowstone.

Then I get up on my creaky knees and hobble to the bathroom.

My weight is our roadblock. We have tempered our dreams. Peru will have to wait. For now it's Greenville.

Even a place like Greenville, on a day as hot as this one, can wear me out. Today, though, I can tell the difference that comes from half a year of exercising and eating better. We have a light lunch at a French place and a little frozen yogurt, and we tote bottles of water around. I feel like I can go all day.

We walk on into the night, doubling back through the downtown streets, ending up at a coffee shop watching a bluegrass band called Conservation Theory. It's the first day in months that I haven't spent any time in a car. My feet are aching by the time we get back to the hotel, but it's a good ache, an earned ache, instead of the hurt of just being fat and old.

On days like this I can see a different life so clearly. I don't have to be limping around, drenched in sweat, scanning around for the nearest bench. Somewhere under all that lard is a pair of strong legs. They can take me to a better place. There are so many rewards for doing it. But there aren't any better than walking around holding hands with the woman I love. She's glowing, she's so happy.

Just before bed, I check the Fitbit. It shows 11,921 steps—a personal record. I can't remember a day when I've been more satisfied. It's the day I'll think of when I try to remember the man I want to be.

Weight on June 30: 444

Weight on July 31: 437

For the month: -7

For the year: -23

Eight

HONESTY IS SUCH A
LONELY WORD

A ll in all, I've done pretty well when it comes to the Ten Commandments. Haven't killed anybody. Never committed adultery. No graven images or false idols. I haven't coveted much—mostly high-end stereo systems and pontoon boats. Only occasionally do I take the Lord's name in vain—usually on Saturdays when my Georgia Bulldogs are losing. When it comes to following the spirit of the commandments, I'd give myself a solid nine out of ten.

One, though, is a real problem.

Thou shalt not lie.

My lust for food has made me a constant liar. I've lied to doctors and coworkers. I've lied to strangers and friends. I've lied to the people who care about me the most. I've told half-truths, left out key facts, spun tales full of bullshit and smoke.

I've done it so nobody but me would know how much I weighed, how much I ate, how much I hated myself for it, how much I wished in those dark moments that everybody would just leave me alone with my addiction.

Mostly, though, I've lied to myself.

My job as a journalist is to find the truth and tell it. My existence as a fat man compels me to run from the truth and hide. I've lived a two-faced life. Which might explain the double chin.

No, Mama, I'm not eating nothin'.

She has come down the hall and peeked around the corner. I'm up late watching TV on the couch. I show her my empty hands. She cuts me a look and goes back to bed. I wait to hear the door close and pull the cookies from my pockets. I turn the pockets inside out to make sure I get the crumbs.

Some version of that scene played out a thousand times in our house. I'd promise not to eat between meals, and then five minutes later I'd shave off a piece of pie while my folks were out working in the garden. I never got whipped or grounded—that was saved for more serious trouble. The only punishment was their disappointment. That hurt worse than anything. It didn't hurt enough to get me to stop.

Most of the time I snuck the food off to my room. I'd be in there doing homework with a bologna-and-cheese when Mama knocked. I'd stash the sandwich in the desk drawer but my tongue always gave me away. I've never been able to stand having food stuck in my teeth. So I'd shake my head *No, I'm not eating right before supper,* and the whole time I'd be running my tongue around my mouth, prying white bread from my molars. She'd call me on it. I'd stick to the lie even though both of us knew better. Mama called lying "telling stories." *God doesn't like it when you tell a story,* she'd say. Sorry, Mama, and sorry, God. By the time I was ten I had a lot of practice at lying about food. You practice anything enough, you get good.

I lied about exercise, too. As a Cub Scout I earned every merit badge I got except one. There was a physical-fitness badge that required tumbling. I couldn't do the rolls on the floor, so I cheated and did them on the bed. In eighth-grade P.E. class, we were supposed to climb a rope to the ceiling of the gym. Just before my turn I'd duck into the bathroom and hide in a stall. (Somehow I had convinced myself this was civil disobedience. I was not exactly Rosa Parks.) Nobody noticed I was gone—everybody was looking up at the kids on the ropes. Or maybe the teachers did notice and they spared me. Either way, there was no way I could pull myself up that rope. I couldn't even pull myself up to the chin-up bar in my bedroom doorway, except for that one time it popped out of the bracket and whacked me in the face.

In high school, the holy grail was sneaking off campus. Some kids did it every day. I was more of a once-a-month guy. I wasn't brave enough to just leave—I'd invent a nonexistent debate-team practice, or something about building the homecoming float. Then I'd go find my fellow truants. The cool kids skipped class to smoke pot or get laid. My group skipped to have lunch at Pizza Inn. That was thirty-five years ago, but we did that buffet so many times I can still remember what it cost: $3.53 with tax. I always left a buck or two extra. When your mama is a waitress, you damn sure better be a good tipper.

When I lived with roommates, I lifted their snacks. I filched Little Debbies and Cheerwine from my friend Zane in college. I peeled off lunch meat from my roommate John Prince's stash in our apartment in Augusta. One morning I woke up to find a note on the fridge. John—as nice a dude as you could imagine—was tired of my thievery: *We have to pull our own weight in this house.* He was completely in the right. But I was never man enough to apologize.

In Jacksonville, where I spent a miserable summer internship, I had one credit card—a Gulf gas card. In my family, credit cards were for emergencies only. One day I asked the cashier at the Gulf station if I could use the card to buy stuff other than gas. Before long I was stopping by there every day to load up on Cheetos and cinnamon rolls and two-liter Cokes and Budweiser. It took just a few weeks to max out the card. My folks paid it off and cut it up. I can't remember what I told them about how I ran up the bill so fast. Whatever I said, it wasn't the truth.

There was one big lie in my career, and although it wasn't directly related to food, maybe in some small way it was.

My last year at UGA, I basically checked out. I cut back my work at the newspaper, then quit. I barely went to class. I didn't have money for a gap year, and I knew I was about to start a lifetime of work. So I arranged my days to be as free as possible. Athens, Georgia, was a tremendous place to float. Five of us lived in that great old run-down house with the ten-foot drop out the back door. I read *Dubliners* on the porch and listened to old Motown on these incredible new inventions called compact discs. I walked down the hill to O'Malley's on Monday nights to drink Milwaukee's Best for a quarter a can. I made love to a girl, nervously, while her dogs tried to claw through the door to the bedroom at her place. I ate burritos for breakfast, burgers at midnight, and takeout all day in between. The delivery guy who brought me ribs one day turned out to be the drummer for one of my favorite bands. This taught me most of what I needed to know about the music business.

At the time I told myself I was having fun, but really I was out of gas, mentally and emotionally and physically. The whole year felt like one long food coma. I didn't have the energy to care. A smart and sexy classmate who lived down the street offered to give me rides to campus in the mornings. More days than not I slept in. This turned out to be stupid, and not just romantically. I needed a C in my last journalism class to get my degree. I made a D.

I ran into the professor on graduation day, and he gave me the news as we were all lining up outside the football stadium for the ceremony. No point in leaving then. The ceremony felt as if it lasted for days. We had a streaker. Champagne bottles wound their way through the rows. Every time a bottle came by, I took a deep pull.

By then, I had already been hired at the newspaper in Augusta. I had filled out the application assuming I would finish my degree. When I got there, nobody asked if I had graduated, and I didn't tell. Three years later, when I applied for the job in Charlotte, I put on my résumé that I had a degree. I started correspondence courses a couple times, intending to make it right. But I never finished. Then something weird happened. In 1994—eight years after I'd left school—the university system of Georgia reduced its requirements for some degrees and made the changes retroactive for ten years. As a result, I backdoored my journalism degree. UGA sent me a diploma. I told my friends about it. Some coworkers threw me a graduation party. It was just a funny story. I didn't even think about the lies I had told.

Three years later, after I'd been promoted to columnist, a local insurance executive and community leader got fired for making up huge chunks of his background—among other things, he'd said he had won an Olympic gold medal in track. I wrote a column about it and mentioned in passing that I had fallen one course short of my degree. The piece made its way up the newsroom chain to the managing editor—Frank Barrows, my mentor, the man who'd hired me as columnist. He killed the column. Only then did it dawn on me that the higher-ups at the paper didn't know I had lied on my application. There were many meetings in the glass offices at the paper, meetings to which I was not invited. My immediate editor, John Drescher, came to my apartment that night with a six-pack. We drank it down and didn't talk much.

The next day I met with Frank and the other two top editors of the paper. They made it clear how serious an offense this was. I apologized every way I knew how. We went over my résumé and job application line by line until they were sure I hadn't made up anything else. They could have fired me. Maybe they should have. Instead they suspended me for a month without pay. I wrote a column telling readers what had happened and apologizing for my lies. I sent notes to my friends. Then I called home to tell my mom what I had done.

That was twenty years ago, and when I think about it I still feel a sick fear in my gut, like I'm about to fall off a roof.

I went home to Georgia for a few days and tried to explain it all to my family. Then I spent a couple weeks driving slowly up the Carolina coast, from Hilton Head to the Outer Banks. The coast always makes me feel better: the waves, the smell of salt, the blue of a tidal creek up against the brown and green marsh grass. That's home.

This is also home: fried shrimp, hush puppies, extra tartar sauce. I stared at the water all day and found a different seafood shack every night. I told myself it was part of the healing process.

Cut to present day.

"Have you had lunch?" Alix asks.

"Mm-hmm," I say, hoping she drops the topic.

"What'd you have?"

Damn.

"A sandwich," I say. This is true, as far as it goes. I am hoping she thinks I made a ham and cheese out of the stuff we have in the fridge, instead of what I actually did, which was get in the car while she was gone and grab a Whopper from the drive-through. There was no good reason to get a Whopper from the drive-through. We have plenty of good food in the house. It was money I didn't need to spend on food I didn't need to eat. But I'm not thinking about any of that right now. I'm trying to decide what to do if she asks what kind of sandwich. Do I give up and tell her the truth, or do I lie?

Part of me really wants her to ask, so I can trade the short-term pain of her disappointment for the long-term satisfaction of being open and honest with the woman I love more than anyone else in the world.

Part of me doesn't want her to ask, because I know what I'll say. Something except the truth.

She moves on. I puff a little sigh of relief and hope she doesn't hear.

Here's an honest thing about lying: There's a thrill to it.

I don't have the guts to lie big, which means I'll never be a great poker player or presidential candidate. I have no desire for a secret life. I don't want to grift or do drugs or keep a woman on the side. I love the life I have. Sneaking off for crappy food when I know better is as close as I get to the shadows.

My worst side surfaces when Alix goes out of town. I'll hit all my favorite spots. Price's Chicken Coop, the best damn fried chicken in the world—I'm no sissy—is fifteen minutes from my house. I almost never go there because it's takeout-only and hard to eat in the car. I always end up with grease on my shirt. But when Alix is gone for a few days, I can bring a box home and the chicken scent will fade before she gets back. I throw the dog some fries to buy his silence.

Then I rearrange the stuff in the fridge so it looks like I ate some of it. Or worse, I *do* eat some of it—a second meal as alibi for the first.

The other day, I knew there was part of a big bag of M&M's in the house, left over from a party. I schemed for days about how to get ahold of them without Alix knowing. I honestly thought about going out and buying *another* bag of M&M's and eating *that* one to soothe my craving.

A day or two later, while I was working, Alix brought me a little handful of M&M's from the bag. Methadone, basically. She knows me well. She loves me anyway. The liar inside me will never get over being surprised at that.

Of all the people I lie to, I'm the easiest to fool.

You know how magicians use misdirection, where they gesture with one hand while they're switching cards or something with the other? That move gets me every time. I can be at a diner, reading a paper or looking at my phone, and a meal will just disappear from my plate. An entire club sandwich or a basket of fish and chips vanishes while I'm not looking. It took years of training to make myself not pay attention when I'm eating something bad. The calories hit my waist but never make it into my brain. Sometimes I'll forget a whole meal minutes after eating it. I'll get a snack on the way home just to taste something I'll remember.

I've learned a million tricks. Watch me cut this slice of cake . . . plus this sliver I eat before I get back to the table. Note how I take a long draw off my Coke while I'm standing at the fountain, then sneak a quick refill. Behold this miracle of balance where I stack a tower of food on a single plate so I can say to myself, *At least I didn't get seconds.*

Consider the layers of deception it takes just to eat a pint of Ben & Jerry's Cherry Garcia: First I have to tell myself that I deserve ice cream. Then I have to tell myself that I deserve Ben & Jerry's Cherry Garcia, instead of all the other very good and much cheaper ice cream at the grocery store. *This is a rare treat. If you're gonna have some, have the best.* Yes! I deserve the best! Then I have to hold the container carefully so as not to see the nutritional info: 1,040 calories, or 260 per half-cup serving, although no one in history has eaten just a half-cup of Ben & Jerry's. Then I have to tell myself it's OK to eat more even though I'm pretty satisfied after three bites. Then (temporary blackout). Then I have to figure out where to hide the empty container.

This suspension of disbelief goes on day after day. I tell myself that a quick stroll around the block is enough exercise, and I believe it. I tell myself that the mound of peanut butter on my sandwich is just a couple teaspoons, and I believe it. I tell myself that a cheat day is just a onetime thing, and I believe it.

The worst lie I tell myself, and the most powerful one, is about tomorrow.

Tomorrow is the golden day. That's the day when I'll quit overeating and start working out and set the course for a new version of myself. Tomorrow means it's OK to eat like a Viking today. Tomorrow means I'd better stuff myself until my stomach hurts, because things are about to change.

It's no different than the lies of alcoholics, or meth addicts, or compulsive gamblers. The lie of tomorrow justifies the same old shit today. Enhances it, even. *Get it out of your system. Carpe diem.*

In acting, the rule about playing a villain is that the villain always thinks he's the hero. Nobody likes to believe otherwise. But I've known for a while now that while I might be a good guy in life, I'm the bad guy in this story. I'll convince myself of just about anything if it lets me keep eating junk food another day. I'm the devil on my own shoulder. The angel is out on break.

I lie to myself more than to everybody else put together. It's how I survive the day. When I look the truth square in the eye, it's too much to handle.

The place where my weight and my lies overlap is shame. I'm ashamed that I'm fat and I'm ashamed of the lies I've told to keep from doing anything about it. The fat is obvious to everyone. The lies weigh me down from the inside.

One night when I was low I wrote a list of everything I could think of that would be better if I lost weight. It goes on for pages and pages. Some of it is simple and shallow. I could ride Space Mountain! (I don't *want* to ride Space Mountain. But it would be great if I *could*.) Some of it is simple and not so shallow; just once, it would be nice if Alix could get her arms all the way around me.

Somewhere on the list I wrote: *I wouldn't lie so much.* In some ways it's more important than losing the weight itself. I believe I'm an honest person. I try to live my life straight up. This is the one place where I'm crooked. I need to bend that bar back right.

I grew up Southern Baptist, in a church so strict we weren't supposed to wear shorts (it was south Georgia, so most of us did anyway). Alix and I now go to a United Church of Christ that prides itself on its diversity in race, sexuality, even belief. I'm a believer with doubts. I tend to think of heaven not as a Hall of Fame, where only the best get in, but as a big unruly bus station where we all eventually find our way home.

One thing I feel sure about is that God hurts when we do wrong. I don't think God would keep me out of heaven for being fat. But every culture I know of condemns lies. If the Lord is a strict constructionist, I'm on shaky ground. I pray for forgiveness. But it keeps me awake some nights. I'm not gonna lie.

AUGUST

I wake up in Las Vegas and it hurts so bad I can barely get out of bed. This is not an uncommon thing in Las Vegas. Most other people get a good story out of it, if they can remember what happened. All I did was throw my back out.

About once a year, my lower back gets tired of hauling my gut around and goes on strike. The muscles turn into overwound guitar strings, right on the edge of popping. This time I just twisted funny in the shower. It hurts to sit down. It hurts to get up. It hurts to walk. It hurts to pee. God help me if I cough or fart or sneeze. Tylenol doesn't even take the edge of the edge off. This is when I see the wisdom of those people who stash a few post-surgery Vicodin for special occasions.

It makes sense that my back would quit now. I've been on the road for work most of the past month—two trips to Syracuse, one to ESPN headquarters in Connecticut, and now this trip. That's seven flights (so far) and a dozen nights in hotel beds. I've gotten a lot of work done, seen a bunch of old friends, and made some new ones. Plus I'm in Vegas and somebody else is paying the bill—that's the definition of blessed. But the airplane seats and strange mattresses have finally caught up to me. I hobble through the Cosmopolitan casino, hunched over and sweating. Every hundred feet or so I stop at a slot machine. I hate slot machines. I just need somewhere to sit for a minute.

I'm doing a story on Syracuse basketball coach Jim Boeheim, who is here as an assistant coach to the U.S. Olympic team. The team is having its first mini-camp at the University of Nevada, Las Vegas. The greatest basketball players in the world have gathered in the practice gym. The first afternoon, these six players run half-court drills in one corner: LeBron James, Steph Curry, Carmelo Anthony, Kevin Durant, Russell Westbrook, and Chris Paul. That squad could beat any team on Earth and possibly other planets. It's breathtaking to watch. I try to enjoy it. But my back ratchets another notch tighter every few seconds. Those of us in the media are watching from a balcony above the courts. There aren't many chairs. Standing is agony. Perching on a bar stool is worse—I don't have anything to lean my back against. So every few minutes I go rest on a couch on the far side of the balcony, away from the action, missing out on the best collection of basketball talent I'll ever see.

Vegas indulges every temptation, and so you can eat anything you want twenty-four hours a day. The big hotels compete for most over-the-top buffet. I try the one at the Cosmopolitan as an experiment: Can I go to a buffet and eat healthy? I stack my plate with baked chicken, a few pieces of sushi, steamed asparagus, and roasted vegetables. I try bone marrow for the first time. Turns out I don't like bone marrow, or at least Vegas buffet bone marrow. I pick a couple of macarons from the half-acre of desserts. I might have eaten less than anyone in the room, including the children. It wasn't a kale salad and water. But it was a victory for me.

Another night, though, I end up with a group of friends at Firefly, a tapas place off the Strip. We drink sangria and order some plates, and keep ordering, and keep ordering. Everything tastes amazing. They have these skewers of steak and chorizo that are just about the best thing I've ever put in my mouth. At the end of the night I try to write down everything I ate for my Fitbit tracking. I know I forgot a few things. Still, I've overshot my calorie limit even though I walked nearly four miles. It's my first blowout day in weeks. I make the walk of shame to the bathroom and wash my face and try to figure out how to make it right. My back throbs, like it's sending me a message in Morse code: *Your back hurts because you eat too much. Idiot.*

There's one other place on my agenda while I'm here. In downtown Vegas there's a restaurant called the Heart Attack Grill. The Heart Attack Grill mocks the idea of healthy eating. They give you a hospital gown when you walk in. The waitresses are sexy nurses. The main menu item is a Bypass Burger—you can get a Double Bypass, Triple Bypass, and so on. The Flatliner Fries are cooked in lard. There's a giant scale outside and another when you walk in, posting your weight in numbers you can see from across the block. If you weigh more than 350 pounds, your burger is free.

With free burgers, as with most things, you pay for what you get. At least one customer has had a heart attack at the Heart Attack Grill. Another regular died of a heart attack while waiting at the bus stop outside. The spokesman for the original restaurant in Arizona died of pneumonia at age twenty-nine. He weighed 575 pounds.

The owner, a former fitness trainer named Jon Basso, makes regular circuits of the cable talk shows to say he is the most honest restaurant owner in the country. He says every fast-food joint in America is killing you—he's just more up-front about it.

Basso comes across as a colossal asshole. It also feels like he's onto something. I watch YouTube videos of people enjoying themselves at the Heart Attack Grill, wolfing giant greasy burgers, getting paddled by "nurses" if they don't finish. They look happy. For doctors and nutritionists and other people who care about what we put in our bodies, this is Dante's ninth circle. But, goddamn, those burgers look good.

I put on my clothes, my back full of knives, and go down to the lobby to get a cab.

For a minute I stand there and watch the crowd around me: grandmothers pulling the slots, guys day-drinking at the bar, couples who might have met fifteen minutes ago heading up to a room.

Most of them will be fine—it's just a getaway, a harmless dance with vice. But for some it is ruination.

I'm drawn to the Heart Attack Grill. But something inside me knows, symbolically or literally, that if I go in there I might not come back out.

I limp around until I find a sandwich shop and get a turkey on wheat. It's not what I want, but it's close enough to what I need. I go upstairs and write a little and go to bed. In the morning, my back feels better.

Weight on July 31: 437

Weight on August 31: 435

For the month: -2

For the year: -25

Nine

THE INVISIBLE WALL

We're all trailed by shadows. They're the conversations our friends and families have about us when we're not around, the things they think but never say to our faces. To see myself better, I need to know what other people see. So I asked.

I emailed a couple dozen friends, asking them a few basic questions: what they remembered about our times together, what they thought about my weight, whether they'd talked to other people about it without me around. Most everybody replied. My mom and my wife sat down separately for longer conversations. In the end I had more than a hundred pages of emails and notes and transcripts that gave me a window into my shadow life.

It took a while to get up the nerve to read it all.

Frank Barrows, my former boss and mentor, remembered a breakfast in Boston. He and his wife were waiting for Alix and me at a journalism conference. I got delayed for some reason, and Alix got there first. She looked at the chairs around the table and frowned. The chairs had arms and she knew they'd be too small for me. She went off and found one that would fit. The three of them didn't talk about it. I got there a few minutes later, none the wiser.

David Duclos, a college roommate and one of my closest friends for more than thirty years, remembered me bringing special diet food to a tailgate at a UGA football game. We met up with David's brother and his friends, who had set out a huge spread. I tossed my food in the trash and ate burgers with them.

Jon Bauer, who roomed with David and me in college, remembered his mother asking if I had a hormonal condition. John Prince and Clint Engel, my roommates in Augusta, remembered seeing a pizza box under my bed. Chris Jones, one of my writer buddies, remembered when we went to spring training together a few years ago. He had worried that I was in pain from squeezing into the seats at the ballparks. (He was right.)

"Someone will ask me how you are doing, which I guess is their way of asking if you have lost weight," said Perry Beard, one of my two oldest friends. "I'll reply that you are about the same."

"It never seems to enter your mind to order the 'diet' plate," said Gainor Eisenlohr, a friend in Charlotte. "I've always wondered if you thought about that."

Several friends were surprised that they don't see me eat more when we go out together. They're baffled at how I'm so much bigger when we all order the same things. They don't see me dive into the fridge when I get home, or stop at the drive-through for a second supper on the way back. Joe Posnanski, my friend for almost thirty years, told *Charlotte* magazine when they profiled me a few years ago: "There's a public Tommy, the parts of him that he lets out. You can see what a funny guy he is and what a good person he is. But I think there are parts of Tommy that he protects."

I built my life that way without knowing it. Some fearful part of me figured that once other people understood the real me, they'd leave.

That has created a distance between me and the people I care about. For years I've longed for the kinds of friendships I read about in books and see in the movies, where people have deep, soul-scraping conversations to help one another through the hardest times. I love my friends and I know they love me, but we just don't talk like that. We get close, rarely, but then we veer off to talk about football or music or work. There have always been unspoken boundaries that none of us cross. Until now I didn't realize that I was the one who drew the lines.

The other thing I didn't fully understand was how much my friends worry about me.

"We wish you could lose some weight because we are worried about your health," David said. "We like you a lot and want you to be around for a long time."

"When you had your heart scare, some of us were almost hoping it would be weight related so you would be motivated to lose weight so you would be healthier," Gainor said.

I worry about them, too. But they have more to worry about. The odds are that I'll be gone before any of them will. That's a terrible burden to put on a friend. With most of my friends, at one time or another, we've stayed up way too late together, drinking or dancing or talking. We specialize in the kind of nights where nothing much happens but you still remember it forever. Back in college, David and I spent a weekend in Atlanta with Perry and Virgil Ryals—my other best friend from seventh grade. The week before we went over, somebody had stolen David's billfold from a dorm shower stall. While we were hanging out in Atlanta, the thief used David's credit card to get a room at a Red Roof Inn across town and trash the place. The cops, of course, thought David had done it. We vouched that he had been with us the whole time. Each one of us had to write an affidavit about what we had been doing that Saturday night. We told the truth: We were eating takeout barbecue and watching *Pee-wee's Big Adventure*.

We were not exactly wild men.

The point is, when you're with the people you love, it doesn't matter what you're doing. You just don't want the night to end. My time with my friends has been one great never-ending party. I don't want to be the first to go home.

Mama is telling me about Marie Osmond's diet plan. She saw it on TV. Marie Osmond says it works. How can you not trust Marie Osmond?

"You'd lose some weight on that," Mama says. "The food's already fixed."

We're sitting at her dining-room table. The two of us have spent untold hours at this table—eating, or talking about eating, or talking about trying to cut back. Mama is in her eighties now and she doesn't cook much anymore unless she's got company. She quit making biscuits after my dad died, because she made so many thousands of biscuits in her life that she got tired of looking at them. But she still makes the best cornbread you will ever put in your mouth. No recipe. She just eyeballs it. Smeared with a little butter, or dipped in the potlikker from some turnip greens, it tastes like home. I could eat a basketful. I have, more than once.

She spent most of her life cooking to take care of her family. These days she lives alone and doesn't see much point in cooking for herself. Lunch might be a slice of bread with some cheese, and maybe mayonnaise and hot sauce. If she has the energy, she might fry an egg and make a little pot of grits. Before I sit down to interview her, we go to Walmart to pick up a few things. She asks me to stop by Taco Bell. She loves a Taco Bell taco. "It's good for you," she says. "It's got lettuce in it."

We talk about Daddy a lot. She remembers him making me homemade french fries as soon as I could eat solid food. She shakes her head at all those times he bought me chocolate milk and crackers at the SeaPak canteen on his way home. It reminds me of all those times I stop at Wendy's on the way home from work. I guess it's the only bad habit he ever taught me. Unless you consider a love of professional wrestling a bad habit. Which I don't.

Whatever bad things he taught me about food mean nothing compared to all the good he taught me. It's the same with Mama. Her big heart taught me how to treat people. Her toughness is with me right now as I try to claw my way out of this mess, even though I'll never be as tough as she had to be. The one thing we can't choose in life is our parents. If I ever got to pick, I'd take the exact same ones.

Mama tells me that she and my dad spent night after night talking about what to do about my weight. They couldn't find a way to help me. "When you went to college, I kept talking to you about it, about your weight. I knew what you was doing. You was sitting around there with them boys hanging around and always eating potato chips, anything that come to hand, and I knew it. Every time you come home you had put on more weight. And I kept saying, 'Tommy, please, slow down on your eating.' You didn't pay me no attention. It was like talking to the side of the house."

That last line makes us laugh. We have always found a way to laugh about the fat in our family. Our sense of humor is part of my inheritance. We've cried about my weight, too, but there's no sense crying all the time.

I remind Mama of a story she told me the last time I was here. Ronald, my brother, had come to visit. He was a star pitcher in high school and college, got drafted by the Baltimore Orioles. He's in his sixties but looks a lot younger. Still, like pretty much everybody else in our family, he's got a belly on him. He and his wife, Neca, spent the night at Mama's house. They asked her not to cook breakfast. In response, she cooked a pound of bacon. He ate just one or two slices at first, but every time he came through the kitchen he grabbed one or two more, and by the end of the day it was gone.

"You didn't have to cook that bacon," I say.

She laughs. "I know I didn't have to."

"He didn't have to eat it, but you didn't have to cook it either."

"Well, I knew they was going to be hungry when they got up."

A mother's logic.

Ronald and I are still her little boys. She is trying her best to take care of us, in the way she took care of her whole family from the time she was twelve. Food is the main thing she can still do to show us her love.

She knows a lot of foods are bad for you. But it's hard for her to see *eating* as bad for you. When she was young and starving, food was survival. When she was older and striving, food was wealth. Now, in her fading days, food is love. These are the things she taught me.

As we talk, it starts to dawn on me: Food was my imaginary friend. I was an only child of sorts, a bookish kid in a blue-collar house. I spent a lot of time alone. That little square of cheese, the first thing in my life I remember: It looked like the sun. That was my light. It scares me to dim that light. Some part of me worries that I'll end up alone again.

If life goes as planned, one day I will go to Mama's funeral, and that will just about ruin me.

But it would ruin her more to go to mine.

Alix and I are talking and the recorder is running. She is remembering the first home project we ever worked on. When we were dating, she bought an unfinished coffee table for her house. She thought working on it would be a fun afternoon for us. We had to sand it before we could seal it. We stood in her backyard and sanded that thing over and over, with finer and finer grains of sandpaper, until my legs started to burn. I went and sat down without really explaining why. It hadn't occurred to her that sanding a table would be too strenuous for me. I didn't have the guts to tell her.

Now I'm trying to explain. "I guess I'm like a little kid," I say now. "If I close my eyes maybe it'll go away."

"And I think that's perfectly natural," she says. "But upon repeated evidence that it's not going away, what are you going to do about it?"

She says this with a smile in her eyes. She teases me about all this every once in a while—never about being fat, but about the doofus logic I come up with sometimes, or the dumb things I do, like dripping salad dressing on my shirt for the ten thousandth time. She has started to drip things onto her shirts, too. I tease her that she is turning into me, which would be a horrible outcome for both of us.

I make her laugh, and there is no sound in the world I love more than her laugh. She thinks I'm handsome, especially when I wear a suit. She appreciates how I treat people. She can lean into me and know I'll hold her steady. One night early in our marriage, just before we went to sleep, she looked at me and said, "You made my life." It was the most important thing anyone has ever said to me. It fuels my heart to this day. I want to live in a way that honors those four words and never makes her feel that she was wrong.

She didn't marry me intending to fix me. But she had no idea it would be so hard for me to fix myself. Before we got married I told her over and over that I would change. We both remember a night at an Applebee's where I told her I had joined the Y and figured out a diet and would get in shape for her, for both of us. This plan had some flaws. First of all, never make any pledges relating to health at Applebee's. Second, I had said the same things countless times to Mama and Daddy and, most of all, myself. Making the promise to Alix should have mattered even more. She chose to spend her life with me.

"You sat me down and said, 'Don't worry, I'm going to take care of this.' And then you didn't," she says. "I felt like that was understandable and it's a hard thing to do. And on the other hand, I felt kind of like you broke a promise."

By and large I've kept the promises I made to her, as she has kept the ones she made to me. We have honored our wedding vows. But I've broken the promise to get healthy so many times that there's nothing left but dust and splinters.

The thing that bugs her the most is when I shut down. She'll suggest something reasonable—a Saturday hike at the lake, maybe—and here's what goes through my mind: *It's so damn hot already; my knee is bothering me; the Georgia game comes on at 3:30; we're going to get eaten up by mosquitoes; she's not even going to want a burger after we're done, we'll just come back home and have a salad with that lite vinaigrette dressing; why do I think this way I hate myself GAAHHHH—*

But I don't say anything. I just look at her blank-faced while a cumulus cloud forms over my head.

That would drive me crazy if I were on the other end.

The thing is, if I just tell her I don't feel like going, we're usually OK. She might persuade me to go anyway, or I might talk her into staying, or we figure out a third way. But instead of playing tennis with her, batting the ball back and forth, I take the ball and bite it in half. I don't know why. Maybe because I don't like conflict. Maybe because I know how silly I'd sound if I said those thoughts out loud.

I've told stories for a living long enough to know that pretty much every story boils down to the same thing: A character you care about struggles to get past an obstacle, trying to reach his or her personal pot of gold. My big obstacle is food. But my struggle with food has created another hurdle that's almost as big—the distance I put between me and the people I love. Alix even has a name for it. She calls it the invisible wall.

The problem isn't just that I can't figure out how to get over or around or through the wall. The problem is that I built the damn thing myself.

My weight has hurt us in a million little ways, and in some deep ways I can never make right.

We tried and tried to have a baby not long after we got married. The natural way didn't work, so we moved to IVF treatments. My part was easy: I went to the fertility clinic and jerked off into a cup, not especially helped by the eighties porn tape they provided. Alix had it harder. Every night for weeks, she stood there and took it as I jabbed a needle into her thigh, injecting her with the hormones that might help us have a child. The odds were against us. We were in our mid-thirties, older than most first-time parents. I had flipped our riding lawn mower a few months before and took a nasty shot to the groin as I fell. There are lots of possible reasons why our hopes died in those petri dishes. One thing I know for a fact is that my sperm count was extremely low, and my sperm were slow and feeble for a man my age. I will always believe it's because I was so fat.

Most of the time we're fine when we're out somewhere and see new parents cradling a baby. Every so often we'll glance at each other and things will get quiet between us. We tell each other it wasn't meant to be. I don't know what was and wasn't. I just know what I did and didn't do.

I have not been the lover she deserves. I get tired too soon. I can't maneuver like a nimbler man. I don't have confidence in my body. There is still something inside me, despite many years of evidence to the contrary, that finds it hard to believe any woman—even my loving wife—would want to sleep with me.

And so I have limited Alix's life because of the limits on mine.

Sometimes she'll plop down and watch TV with me instead of exercising, because she wants to spend time with me however she can get it. She has gained a few pounds she never would have gained if not for me. When we do go for a walk, sometimes she turns her ankle because she walks so close to the edge of the sidewalk. She walks along the edge because I take up so much space. She could walk so much faster than I do, but she lingers so we can walk together. Part of me wants her to go on ahead. Part of me worries that one day she will just leave me behind.

Our house is not as nice as she'd like because I get exhausted just thinking about painting our bedroom or digging a flower bed. We haven't traveled like we told each other we would. When we do travel, sometimes I get so worked up about how far we have to walk or where I'm sitting on the plane that it's not fun for either of us. When she asks me how she can help, I shut down again.

"I think when we—you—make decisions whether or not to do things, you're making your decisions partly out of fear," she says. "Because as you go out into the world, you run into situations over and over again where some random person will make a crack out of your weight out of the blue . . . and it leads you to make decisions out of fear about what you'll do or where you'll go and what kind of things you're going to do. Because over and over again, it's been proven somewhat unpredictable when you're going to encounter that negative response. And so you—I think you withdraw a little bit and sort of in a way self-censor what you're doing."

It's bad enough when I don't even try to eat right or exercise. The worst part is when I use my size as a reason to close the door on everything else. I assume I can't do something, or I think it'll be too hard, so I never give it a shot. And so both of us delete another item from the mental list of the life we hoped to have together.

She says: "I've had to do some work on my own outlook and my own thinking in terms of what do I expect from a relationship, and what do I expect from another person, and where does my self and their self begin and end, and what's reasonable to expect. Where do I need to say this is about me and not about you?"

I say: "Do you feel like you've gotten less than you hoped for?"

She says: "No. I think it's all to the good. It's all been much more than I had ever dreamed. I just didn't know the best questions to ask beforehand to understand more fully what I was getting into."

I used to give Alix nightmares. In the nightmares I died from something preventable, something that never would've happened had I lost weight like I promised. She was there in the dream alone, a young widow. She would wake up angry and scared.

One of the ways I know I'm slowly getting better is that she's not having those nightmares anymore.

But we both worry about how much longer we have together. Her grandfather lived to be 101. She's got great genes. If I don't turn things around, she's facing a long stretch of years after I'm gone. We have given each other our blessing to find another if one of us dies. We know the chances are she'll need that blessing more than I will.

Most of the time we talk about these things in bits and pieces. It's hard to talk about them all at once. Weeks later, when I read the transcripts of the conversations we recorded, I noticed the kindness of the person who typed them up. When Alix and I laughed, the transcriptionist wrote it down: (Laughter). When we cried, all it said was: (Pause).

Most days I think I'm the laughter in Alix's life. Some days I worry that I'm just the pause.

This, most of all, is what keeps me trying. She deserves the best of me. She made my life, too.

When I'm needing signs of hope, sometimes I look at our old coffee table, the one Alix bought to mark our new life together. We finished it eventually, and it has now lived with us in three different houses and one apartment. It's been the centerpiece of our living room the whole time we've been married. The edges are dented and chipped. But run your hand across the top and it feels as smooth as it was the day we sanded it. We worked hard on it and made it into a beautiful thing. It's built to hold up.

SEPTEMBER

Our terrible month starts with a few drops of blood on a towel.

Alix took Fred with her to visit her parents while I was on the road for work. When she got back home, she noticed blood on the towel she had draped over the backseat for Fred to sleep on. Then, when they got in the house, he sneezed and sprayed blood all over the bedroom floor.

We make an appointment with our vet. She doesn't find anything. But she suggests we take him to a specialist where they can do a more thorough ultrasound.

They find something.

Fred has a big tumor, four by five inches, clinging to his liver. It's most likely cancer. They could do surgery. But there might be more tumors in places the ultrasound can't see. And in his condition—feeble, arthritic—the operation might kill him. He's fourteen years old, ancient for a Lab. Even if the surgery works, chances are he won't make it to fifteen.

So we talk about it and cry about it. And in the end, we decide not to do the surgery.

We had been married just three years when Fred showed up at

the end of our driveway one morning, a stray puppy bloated with worms and crawling with fleas. He was so happy to see us. We didn't have a fence, so we took him across the street to our neighbors' house while we figured out what to do. As we were walking back, he showed up right on our heels. He had squeezed through their gate. We had a dog.

Our old house had a huge backyard. I'd let him wander back there in the mornings while I waited by the corner of our garden. After a few minutes I'd whistle for him and hold up a treat, and he'd take off running toward me. Watching him run that fifty-yard dash every morning, sliding past me as he jammed on the brakes, bouncing with joy when I reached down and scratched his ears, is something I'll take with me until the day I die. I've never seen such beauty.

He got old and it snuck up on us. When he was young he would pull us around the block on walks. Then he walked beside us. For the last year or two, he has trailed behind. Now we sometimes have to lift him when he can't get up by himself. He breathes heavy and hard in the night. To us, it all happened gradually. But when our vet sees him, after a gap of just a few months, she's shocked at how much he has declined. After we go to the specialist, we come back to our vet and tell her about the tumor. She says we should pick a day and put him to sleep. At this point, no day would be wrong.

We pick a day in early October and pray he lasts that long.

Not long after that, on a Saturday morning, I get an email from ESPN human resources. It says they've learned that I'm leaving the company—in classic corporate-speak, they call it *off-boarding*—and that I should get my paperwork in order before I go. I figure it must be a mistake. My contract is up in November, but I haven't heard anything but good things about my work. I leave messages for my editor and her boss, letting them know about the email but sort of laughing about the whole thing.

That afternoon I get a call from my boss's boss. The first thing he does is apologize for the way I found out.

He says he's trying to save my job, but ESPN is having to make budget cuts across the board. The end of my contract falls right at the time they need to cut. They still like my work. He says it's mostly bad timing. But he can't tell me if they'll be able to renew my contract. I hang up the phone and just sit there for a while, poleaxed.

Journalism has shed tens of thousands of jobs over the past decade. Some of the best writers, editors, designers, and photographers I know are scrambling for jobs or have settled for some other field where they have steady work and benefits. It's been just two years since I got let go by Sports on Earth. This time the stakes are higher, because Alix left her job at the paper in April. Right now she has some clients as a coach. But she's still building the business. My deal with ESPN is part-time, but it's my biggest contract and my steadiest work—and the people I work with are some of the best in the business. If I get let go, it's going to hurt bad.

We are still grieving over Brenda, and heartbroken about Fred, and stressed about my job. The life we built feels as if it's falling out from under us.

I take Fred for walks and try to talk it out. He's mostly deaf, too, so he's not much help. The one language he still knows is treats. Our neighborhood has a lot of dogs, so the neighbors down the street started leaving a water dish and a jar of treats on the sidewalk. Fred doesn't want to walk far anymore but he always wants to make it to the treat jar. I reach in and grab him three or four. In the shape he's in, he deserves something good in his life.

When we get home, I dive into my own treat jar—peanut butter and crackers, mostly. I quit wearing my Fitbit for a few days. It takes all my strength to stay away from Wendy's. At the end of the month I step on the scale at the Y, thinking I've probably gained ten pounds. I'm surprised at the number. Maybe stress is a good diet plan.

Weight on August 31: 435

Weight on September 30: 435

For the month: no change

For the year: -25

Ten

THE MAN WHO WALKS
INSIDE ME

There's a man who walks beside me, he is who I used to be

And I wonder if she sees him and confuses him with me.

—Jason Isbell, "Live Oak"

O ne of my biggest fears about losing weight is that I'll end up thinner and healthier but a worse human being.

I've never been anything but fat. I've never lived with any other version of myself. What if I just end up obsessing about something else? What if the switch I have to flip to lose weight turns me from a nice guy into an asshole?

That's not rational. Of course it's not rational. But if this were a rational subject I wouldn't weigh four bills to begin with.

That Jason Isbell song "Live Oak" hits me so hard. The narrator is a killer who falls in love with a good woman and sees a glimmer of a better life for himself. But he wonders which version of him she's attracted to: the one who's trying to live straight now, or the rogue in his past. The song does not have a happy ending.

Isbell is an alcoholic whose addiction nearly ruined his life. The people who loved him had an intervention and sent him to rehab. Now he's clean and making brilliant music; I think he's the best living writer in America right now. But while he was getting sober, he worried about the pieces of himself he was casting off. He said in one interview with Lehigh Valley Music: "I was thinking, when I get my life sorted out and stop behaving irrationally, am I going to lose something, you know? Is there something that people are drawn to that's going to be left behind? And are there really two people there—the person I am now and the person I was before?"

That's what I wonder, too. Is there something in the fat version of me that also makes me likable and creative and a decent human being? Are the best parts of me all knotted up with the worst? Is there some way to untangle it and leave just the good stuff behind?

Most of the time I think of my fat as a husk—something I have to shed so the best part of me can come out. But sometimes I wonder if I'm more like the shells I used to find on the beach, where the outer part is the attraction, and the animal inside is dull and shapeless.

My story is "Live Oak" inside out. There's a man who walks inside me. He is who I'm going to be. I hope when people meet him, they don't prefer the other me.

I can hear what you're thinking: *You're not going to be fat anymore? How awful! You mean it won't wear you out to walk up a flight of stairs? You can flop down in a chair and not worry about it? You'll be able to buy a shirt at the mall? You might live twenty extra years? How terrible!*

There's no doubt. If I wrote down everything that will be better when I lose weight, it would be as long as the Old Testament. If I wrote down everything that might get worse, it wouldn't fill up an index card.

But this is why people buy insurance—to hedge against unlikely disasters.

I've always felt like I needed to lead with my mind and my heart because my body wasn't going to make anybody notice—except in a bad way. Has struggling with my fat been the thing that's kept me sharp? Will I lose some of that edge if I'm not struggling so much anymore?

What's my true identity?

I'm not dumb enough to think that losing weight will cleanse me of self-doubt. All I'm hoping is that it shaves off the lowest of the low, when it feels like the only thing that matters in the world is the meal in the bag on the seat of my car.

Those black thoughts don't happen often. They happened enough to worry me, for a time, when I was covering all those murders and disasters for the paper. The darkness of what I was writing about blended with the darkness I saw inside myself, and it caved in over me. I saw a therapist for a while. She used a method called EMDR, or eye movement desensitization and reprocessing. I would stare at a dot moving back and forth across a screen, listening to a series of beeps, until I felt ready to talk. This was supposed to reduce my anxiety. Most of the time it felt like a goofy gimmick. I'd just start talking to quit having to stare at the dot. But when I did start talking, I ended up crying a lot. And no matter where we started, I ended up in the same place: Because I was so fat and couldn't control it, I felt worthless. After a few months I dug myself out far enough to see a little light. For the most part I've felt better since.

Thank you, goofy-ass dots.

Of course I'm worthy of love. That's always been true. But it took a long time to say it out loud, and until this very moment for me to write it down.

Thinking about all this makes me want it to happen faster.

I've set out on this slow road on purpose. Quick fixes have never worked for me. Based on the research I've read and my own experience, it makes sense to taper down. I'm trying to fool my body into thinking I'm not on a diet at all. I believe in the idea. Then I start itching to speed things up. That's when the Whole30 diet starts whispering my name. *Thirty days,* it purrs, in Kathleen Turner's voice. *All I need is thirty days . . .*

That's our nature as human beings, and definitely as Americans. We'll sacrifice most anything for speed and convenience. When researchers noticed that cereal sales were going down, they did a study to figure out why. It turns out millennials don't eat as much cereal because *it's too much trouble to wash the bowl.* They grab protein bars or yogurt cups and scarf them on the way to work. Cooking shows are more popular than ever—you can find Bobby Flay putting meat on a fire twenty-four hours a day—but it seems like people are watching instead of cooking, in the same way people watch *Fixer Upper* a lot more than they fix anything up. The proof is on the shelves. The stuff you used to find in the 7-Eleven is now in the grocery store: Lunchables, protein packs, quickie meals packed in plastic clamshells. Life, to go.

(This might be the time to launch the idea I've been thinking about awhile: inconvenience stores. They have the very best stuff at great prices, but they're way out in the country, and the shelves are through a maze of hallways and down a few flights of stairs. You can't order online. They don't even have a phone. I'm guessing this will not pose much of a threat to Amazon.)

There is a welcome countercurrent to all the quick meals and quick fixes. The Slow Food movement, designed to get people to cook at home again, is building around the country. Farmers' markets and homemade goods are catching hold in the suburbs. It's along the lines of the new craving for music on vinyl, where the materials matter and you have to get up and flip the record instead of streaming forever. Some of those slower, smaller, more personal ideas are starting to seep into how we take care of ourselves. Atul Gawande, the surgeon and writer, talks about the difference between health and well-being. Terminal patients who have lost nearly all their health can still find pockets of well-being that make their lives worthwhile. Gawande writes about one patient who was facing a severe disability and said he could put up with a lot of pain if he could still eat ice cream and watch football. I'm thinking about my life the same way: What do I need to be happy that makes the slow struggle of losing weight worth it? In the end, it's not much. I need family and friends. Good live music. Time near the water. And, yeah, some ice cream and football, too.

Overcoming any addiction means something else has to fill that space. I like to play poker—every time I go to a city with a casino, I try to get in a few hours at the tables. Sometimes I look around in the middle of a game and I see a lifer: dead-eyed, fish-belly skin, one of those guys who has surely drawn to an inside straight with his rent money. And I wonder: Did he always need the action? Or did he give up something else, and the action took its place?

This is the big question for the man who walks inside me. Once I kill the hog, will I be fine? Or do I need to be hooked on *something*? There's only one way to know.

I'm already preparing for when the man who walks inside me comes to stay.

There are some clothes I want him to wear. In the bottom drawer of my dresser is a stack of T-shirts that are too small for me now. There's one for Willie's Wee-Nee Wagon, the greatest restaurant in the world. There's one for St. Paul and the Broken Bones, one of my favorite bands. There's one for Rapala fishing lures that's so old I can't remember where I got it. It's an XL—five sizes smaller than what I wear now. If the day comes when I can wear an XL shirt, I'll go to my favorite bar—Thomas Street Tavern in Charlotte—and buy a round for the house.

There's a ladder I want the man who walks inside me to climb—the pull-down ladder to our attic. It's rated at 250 pounds. I've never been up in the attic because I'm afraid the ladder won't hold me. Whenever we need what's up there—Christmas ornaments, winter clothes, an extension cord—Alix has to go up and get it. I'm embarrassed that there's an entire part of our house that I've never been in. I want to climb that ladder with confidence.

There's a boat I want the man inside me to put in a lake. Daddy's johnboat lives in our backyard. It's green aluminum and still has its Georgia registration number on the side. When I was a kid we hauled a thousand catfish over the side of that boat. Daddy died in 1990 and the boat hasn't been in the water since way before then. I've always been afraid that I'm so big I'd tip it over. It needs a drain plug and a little love. But it's still strong enough to hold a normal-sized man, and maybe his beautiful wife.

There's a place I want the man inside me to go. My friend Jon Bauer moved to Japan not long after college and never moved back. He got married and teaches English in Hamamatsu, on Japan's southern coast. He posts beautiful pictures from there on Facebook. I've always thought Japan would be impossible for me—all those tiny hotel beds, all those crowds shoved together on the Tokyo subway. I want to move in that world without everyone thinking I'm a sumo wrestler.

There's a bicycle I want the man inside me to ride. Nothing fancy—I'd be fine with one of those old-man bikes with straight handlebars and a cushy seat. Our neighborhood is full of bike riders. There's a group that rides through the neighborhood every Tuesday night. Sometimes we sit on the porch and wave at them as they glide past our house, a rolling parade. I'm tired of watching parades. I'd like to be in a few.

There's a game I want the man inside me to play. Damn, I miss basketball. It's been so long since I boxed out for a rebound or put up a shot with a hand in my face. It doesn't matter if I'm just the old guy who jacks up threes from the corner. It doesn't matter if I sprain my ankle for the eighteenth time. It would feel so good to be back in the game again.

There's a flight I want the man inside me to take. It doesn't matter where it goes as long as I'm in the middle seat. I want to sit there without flooding the banks of the armrests. I want the seat belt to click around my waist with an inch or two to spare. After that, I can bitch about the middle seat like everybody else. But I'd like to sit there and feel good about it. Just once.

My favorite wrestler growing up was Dusty Rhodes. He was brilliant on the microphone—Huey Long plus Muhammad Ali with a toke of Willie Nelson. His dreaded Bionic Elbow (pretty much his only move) took down all his opponents, especially the hated Ric Flair. The best thing about Dusty was that he wasn't one of the pretty boys. He had a scarred forehead, and a giant weird birthmark, and a gut that hung down over his tights.

One of the wrestling magazines I read as a kid did a story on Dusty's strengths and weaknesses, like an NFL scouting report. The story listed one of his strengths as his "rim of flesh." The idea, apparently, was that his extra padding cushioned him from the bumps every wrestler takes. His fat was his shield.

It took me a long time to see it, but I've used my rim of flesh the same way. I've forged my weight into a shield that keeps me from the risks of a bolder life. I won't try things because I think I'm too fat, when maybe the truth is that I'm fat because I don't want to try things. I'm a more boring person than I ought to be. The chance to be more interesting is slipping away, and I've convinced myself that it's OK.

It's not OK.

I've shielded my feelings the same way. It's easy to write off people who don't like me—I can always tell myself it's because I'm fat. But what if I'm not fat anymore, and they still don't like me? That's a laser through the shield. And I worry that I'm soft underneath.

Thinking this way is borrowing trouble, I know. It's dumb to worry about something that might never happen. It's even dumber to let that worry get in the way of changing for the better. The fact is, I've got two options: Lose weight and expose myself to some theoretical risk, or stay the way I am and walk straight for the grave.

I've never met the man who walks inside me. I don't know what people will think about him. But if I want to live, I've got to find out.

OCTOBER

We lift Fred up onto our couch, me at his head, Alix at his feet. Our vet, Dr. Mary Fluke, pulls up a chair next to us. She has taken care of him since he was a puppy. She cries as she opens her medical bag. It's time.

We gave him a good last week. We found out near the end that he liked tuna, and in those last days it was about all he would eat.

He devoured a can every meal. He also started farting loudly and le-thally. Maybe it's good we didn't figure out the tuna thing right away.

He didn't want to walk far. Some days he'd wander out into the yard and just stand there. One of us would pick him up—we bought a vest with handles to make him easier to lift—and tote him back to the house. But on his next-to-last day, he went down to the corner where we usually turned around and pulled me ahead one more block. It felt so good to see the headstrong dog we used to know.

On one of those last nights I took him out for his midnight pee and we came back and sat on the top step of the porch. Alix came out to join us and he put his head in her lap, and if I had to freeze time forever, never moving from one spot, that's where I would stay.

His last meal is bacon. I lie down next to him on his dog bed and we both fall asleep. We give him one more car ride, rolling the window down and letting him feel the breeze. Dr. Fluke comes. We tell Fred how much we love him. We thank him for finding us.

Dr. Fluke does her work and soon he is quiet, and soon after that he is still.

That weekend Alix and I go to the beach to clear our heads. It rains the whole way and we get crossways at the hotel. But we make up and take a walk on the beach even though it's still raining. We get soaked and look terrible and laugh for the first time in days.

Back home, though, I can't get traction. I try to write and can't find the words. I keep looking for Fred to come around the corner, keep wondering why he's not sleeping at my feet. When I feel the worst I go back to my worst habits. One day's lunch: two Whoppers with cheese, a family-sized bag of Utz chips, a large Coke, and a sleeve of Chips Ahoy. That's not falling off the wagon. That's diving off the wagon, rolling down a mountain, and plunging into a bottomless lake.

We go out of town for Halloween, and that's good. Our street gets trick-or-treaters from three or four nearby neighborhoods. The first year we lived here, Alix had to make two runs to the CVS to buy enough candy. Now we load up on army-sized bags from Costco. Normally on Halloween night I test the candy—for quality-control purposes, of course—and end up eating three of everything. This year we remove ourselves and remove the temptation.

But Fred is still gone, and I still try to fill the empty space with food. It never works that way.

Weight on September 30: 435

Weight on October 31: 439

For the month: +4

For the year: -21

Eleven

USUCK-FM

A few years ago I wrote a story about a guy my size—well, almost my size—named Jared Lorenzen. Jared was a record-setting quarterback at the University of Kentucky in the early 2000s, slinging bombs even though he weighed nearly three hundred pounds—bigger than many of his linemen. Fans called him the Hefty Lefty. After three years as a backup in the NFL, he drifted. When he popped up on TV in 2014, the anchors on *SportsCenter* were making fun of him. He was still playing football, earning two hundred dollars a game for an indoor-league team called the Northern Kentucky River Monsters. He was wearing a ridiculous green jersey that clung to him like sharkskin. He had grown to somewhere around four hundred pounds—nobody knew exactly, because he refused to get on a scale. He was the biggest player on the field and surely the biggest quarterback ever to play in a professional game.

I watched the clip and saw a story. I called him up and went to his home in Lexington, Kentucky, and talked to him fat guy to fat guy. We understood each other immediately. Here's the beginning of the piece I wrote for *ESPN The Magazine*:

> *Jared Lorenzen and I are in love with the same woman. Her name is Little Debbie, and she makes delicious snack cakes. We're not the only ones who love her. Nick Saban has two Oatmeal Creme Pies every morning for breakfast. I'm more of a Nutty Bars man myself. "They're all right," Lorenzen says. "But I'll kill a Fudge Round."*
>
> *We bond over clothes from Casual Male XL. It's the only place we can walk into and find stuff that fits. I wear a 6X shirt. Lorenzen is a 4XT—T for tall, because he's six-foot-four. He says he's usually a 3X. That's a classic big-guy line—*This size is just temporary. *"My pants are a 54, but that's because my thighs are so damn big,"* he says. *"I have to cinch my belt way down or my pants fall off."*

The piece ended up being one of ESPN's most-viewed stories of 2014. Millions of people read it. Tens of thousands shared it on Facebook and Twitter. Hundreds of readers sent me letters. Some people shared intimate stories about their own struggles with weight. Others said they had a new understanding of what it's like to battle the temptation to overeat. For years, I'd been afraid to write about my own life as a fat guy. Writing about Jared helped me figure out a way. Reading those letters made me see it might mean something to other people. If not for that story, I wouldn't have written this book.

Jared has a better sense of humor about his weight than I do.

Another of his nicknames as a QB was the Pillsbury Throwboy, so he started a T-shirt company called Throwboy Tees. But he's still struggling with his weight.

Every story I've done lives with me a little. Jared's lives with me more than most. There's one part I think about a lot. He was talking about his relationship with Tamara, the love of his life and mother of their children. They had been together eighteen years and married for six. They still cared for each other, but they got tired of arguing over Jared's weight. A few months before we talked, they had gotten a divorce.

"We're best friends," he said. "She's awesome. But being divorced, that got me where it's just chomp-chomp-chomp-chomp. *Who do I have to live for?* Chomp-chomp-chomp."

That's the moment it hit me. Jared had the same radio station playing in his head that I've been hearing my whole life.

USUCK-FM.

The great writing teacher Chip Scanlan was the first one I heard put a name on it. It's that voice that tells you you're not good enough, the voice that wonders why you ever believe in yourself, the one that leans in your ear when you're facedown on the ground and tells you you're a failure. The voice is low and relentless. There are no ads on USUCK-FM and no music. There are only public service announcements. *There's no point. You'll never make it. Don't even try.*

That voice is the distillation of my craving and my lying and my anger and my shame. It's the sound of the salt grinding in my arteries and the grease hardening my heart. It is the careless whisper of death, telling me it's fine to give in and give up.

There are times when it fades—when I write a story that moves people, when I'm laughing with family and friends, when Alix and I are tangled together in bed. But every time I let down for a second, USUCK-FM comes back in high definition. It never takes a day off.

It's hard for me to write with music in the background—I end up tapping the beat with my fingers instead of typing. But silence is worse. USUCK-FM fills the empty space. This is why I know that YouTube has multiple videos of nothing but a box fan running for ten or twelve hours straight. This is why I can tell you the YouTube box fan that provides just the right hum of white noise. There's no mute button on USUCK-FM. You have to drown it out.

When I was a teenager, USUCK-FM told me no girl would ever like me. When I was right out of school, it told me I'd never be good at my job. These days it tells me I peaked ten years ago.

It saves its most ruthless chatter for the times I try to get in shape. It reminds me of all the times I've tried before and quit. It tells me there's something broken inside me that can't be fixed. It tells me to go ahead and finish off that pizza, because it doesn't make any difference.

I used to wonder: Does anybody else hear that? Then I learned that many of us have our own personal station, customized to punch us in the kidneys the moment we start to feel good about ourselves. I haven't met many people who never hear that voice. Some of the people who act the most confident, I've found, are the ones who hear it the loudest.

USUCK-FM is a cousin to impostor syndrome—the idea that

you're a fraud and will eventually be found out. It's a common psychological problem, especially among high achievers. Even Albert Einstein had it. Late in life, in a letter to Queen Elisabeth of Belgium, he wrote: "The exaggerated esteem in which my lifework is held makes me very ill at ease. I feel compelled to think of myself as an involuntary swindler." When I worked for the *Charlotte Observer*, our legendary sports columnist Ron Green retired after working there fifty years. At his retirement party, I told him I admired how he wrote so well for so long. He said: "Every day I came to work, I thought that was the day they were going to fire me."

Steven Pressfield, in the book *The War of Art*, lumps the forces of self-sabotage into one thing he calls Resistance, and he believes it's an actual evil presence, like the devil. What scares me about that idea is that I don't hear some satanic cackle when USUCK-FM is on. What I hear is my own voice. It's me not believing in me. The call is coming from inside the house.

The result of all this is that my life has fewer colors in it. I plow my little fields deeply but don't wander off much. I end up watching things more than doing them. When I teach journalism classes, I always tell students to live a full life—even if they don't write about it, the experiences and emotions will work their way into the stories. I'm terrible at following my own advice.

In some ways I know USUCK-FM is just the voice of fear. Fear has it harder than it used to. Most of us are lucky enough that we don't have to face life or death every day—the commute to work no longer involves bears trying to eat us. So those old useful fears spread into places they don't belong. They morph into anxieties and superstitions and phobias. Instead of just keeping us alive, they keep us from being our best.

In other people I know, USUCK-FM takes much darker forms. One friend of mine has dealt with depression since he was a child. He can't remember ever having a happy day. Despite that, he has a beautiful family and has built a towering career. The older I get, the more I'm in awe of people who have to climb out of such a deep hole every day just to get anything done. Even on my worst days, when the voice is blaring the loudest, I can still see up above the rim.

The thing I have always wanted to know about USUCK-FM is why. Where does that voice come from? Why does it pull me toward the worst version of myself? What does it want from me?

My old calendars are littered with broken promises. Here's when I started that diet. Here's when I vowed to start going to the gym every Wednesday and Saturday. Here's where I wrote in my journal that this was the LAST time I'd ever touch fast food, so help me God. Here's a Seinfeld chain, from Jerry Seinfeld's idea that if you want to get good at something, you have to do it every day. Look at the row of X's marking off every day that I met my goals. Look how they disappear after a week or two. This is the maddening part. I knock USUCK-FM to the floor, broken and beaten, and then I let him up every time.

The easiest thing to call it is laziness, or a lack of willpower. In my case, I could also blame all the forces lined up against my effort to lose weight: all the easy and cheap junk to eat, all the entertainment to keep me planted in my chair, all the advertising calibrated to make me keep craving the very foods that hurt me.

All those things are true, and if you want to claim any of them for your own, I hear you. But they never felt like the answers for me.

One night after another eating binge I lay in bed sleepless, Alix breathing deep beside me. A new voice came into my head. It sounded like me, too. But it wasn't USUCK-FM. It was trying to help.

Why do you do this to yourself? it said.

I don't know, I said. Maybe I want to die.

You know that's not true. Go deeper.

I don't want the ones I love to die before me.

Go deeper.

I don't want to be alone.

Deeper.

I don't want to get old. Being old looks too hard.

Almost there.

I don't want to grow up.

That's it.

That's it.

I stole my own childhood from myself. I ate and ate and ate and so I never jumped off a high dive, never sprinted across a football field, never played spin the bottle at a party. I missed out on so much I can never get back. So something deep inside of me refuses to grow up.

Grown-ups watch what they eat. Grown-ups exercise. Grown-ups stick to a schedule. Grown-ups are honest with other people and with themselves. The boy inside me says: *Fuck that.*

I stare out into the dark. I can hear Alix breathing soft and slow. I ought to wake her up to apologize. She thought she married a man, but instead she got this child who can't control his worst impulses. She doesn't deserve this. Yet she chooses me every day and sleeps beside me every night.

She has this amazing talent of being able to fall asleep within seconds of closing her eyes. One night we were talking in bed and she reached out, caressed my face . . . and then she was out cold, her hand still draped over my eyes. Sometimes I tell that story for a laugh. But it has come to mean so much more. That peaceful sleep of hers, knowing what she knows about me. That hand resting on my face instead of pulling away. She feels the good inside me that sometimes I can't feel. She loves me when I can't figure out how to love myself. Her heart is the truest thing I know. There, in the dark, I have never wanted anything more than just to be her man.

One Sunday not long after that restless night, Nancy Allison—our pastor at Holy Covenant United Church of Christ—preached a sermon that felt like she had been listening to my thoughts. "How many of us," she said, "even into our thirties or forties or fifties, say, 'When I grow up . . .' or 'In my next life . . .'? It's a way of minimizing our existence. Of asking people—God—not to expect too much of us today."

It made me think of something I'd written in my Jared Lorenzen story: "Part of being an adult is taking care of your body. He and I agree that we can't be grown men until we are not such overgrown men."

In much of my life I'm a grown-ass man. I work for a living, pay taxes, cut the grass, follow the news, vote. But underneath all that I want to be a kid. I want to stay up late and sleep in. I want to lie around and watch TV. When I moved to Charlotte as a single man, I bought a video game console—it was long enough ago that the hot console was a Sega. It came with a Tiger Woods golf game. I bought it on a Friday and played all weekend. I mean ALL weekend. On Monday I took it back to the store. I couldn't have the thing in the house, because if I did, that's all I'd do.

Looking back, it's amazing how many ways I've dodged adulthood. I've never had a job where I had to punch a clock. I write a lot of sports, which most definitely has grown-up issues, but at its core is people playing kids' games for fans who jump up and down in the stands. I didn't have younger brothers or sisters. Alix and I don't have children. I've never had to be responsible for anyone except our dog.

Lew Powell, a great writer for the *Observer*, once said that the surest sign of an adult is the ability to accept delayed gratification. When it comes to food, I want to be gratified NOW. Alix can tell when I'm stressed at meals because I try to stuff everything in my mouth at once. Whenever I get ice from the freezer, I always grab too big a handful and drop a couple cubes on the floor. It pisses me off every single time, as if I just now realized what would happen. This is not how an adult behaves.

One of my favorite procrastination tricks is to read about the habits of successful people. What I see, over and over, is discipline. Successful people are always getting up at five in the morning to go to the gym. They cook and freeze a week of meals in advance.

They block out times for reading, TV watching, even sex. They don't waste time. Anthony Trollope, the nineteenth-century British writer, wrote for three hours every morning before going to his job at the post office. If he finished a book with ten minutes left in his three hours, he grabbed a blank sheet of paper and started the next book. He wrote forty-seven novels that way, plus many volumes of short stories and nonfiction. That's how a grown-up gets it done.

I'm not Trollope. Some days I watch cartoons and eat Doritos all day. But finally, after all these years, I'm starting to understand why. The child inside you never goes away. The child inside *me* rages at having to be responsible. He is eternally unsatisfied because he never was wild and free. The most dangerous thing he ever did was eat too much. So he roots around in my dreams and whispers in my ear, nudging me to touch the fire again.

I was reading back through the Jared Lorenzen story the other day and came across a passage that I wrote but had forgotten:

> *So much of loving sports comes from connecting with your inner child—the one who revels in the sheer joy of the game and the one who spits and hollers and stays up all night. But here's the conflict: At some point, in sports and in life, you have to quit giving in to everything the kid wants. The inner child doesn't understand that you can't eat pizza every day, in the same way it doesn't understand that you can't throw touchdowns forever.*

I can't be a grown man until I'm not such an overgrown man.

That hog from my dream, the beast I've been trying to kill

all this time? It's the evil Peter Pan in me, the boy who won't grow up.

I can't kill him. But to live the life I want—to live any kind of life at all—I have to quiet him down.

Every day I eat right, every day I exercise, I reach closer to the off switch on USUCK-FM. I finally feel like I have the power. I want to grow up.

NOVEMBER

Thanksgiving is the ultimate cheat day. A lot of modern diets have cheat days, where you eat whatever you want so you don't feel deprived when you're eating cabbage soup the rest of the week. Thing is, my whole life has been a cheat day. So most of the time, Thanksgiving hasn't felt out of the ordinary. Different grub, same calories. My Fitbit gives me a low battery warning when we wake up Thanksgiving morning. I'm pretty sure it's hoping to die by the afternoon so it doesn't have to witness the carnage.

We're in east Tennessee, where Alix's folks moved after they retired. Our hosts for Thanksgiving dinner are Alix's cousin Jeff and his wife, Kathie. Jeff recently had surgery for prostate cancer. Kathie had leukemia and needed a stem cell transplant to save her life. They made it through and their sense of humor survived. When we walk in, Jeff is wearing an apron with the Los Pollos Hermanos logo from *Breaking Bad*. Just to be clear: Our Thanksgiving dinner does not include meth.

However, sweet baby Jesus, it includes just about everything

— 215 —

else. The platters hang over the edge of the kitchen table. There might be one or two dishes a nutritionist would recommend—I see beets over in the corner—but otherwise it's a homemade Golden Corral: turkey and ham, dressing and mashed potatoes, mac 'n' cheese and green bean casserole. Gravy to pour over everything. An olive tray to fill in any exposed areas on your plate. You want full coverage on Thanksgiving.

Getting seconds on Thanksgiving is required by the Constitution. I also have pecan pie with a shot of whipped cream for dessert. But this is a fast compared to my normal Thanksgiving haul. In the old days I would've stacked food on my plate vertically as much as horizontally. It was quite a feat of engineering, like Richard Dreyfuss making Devils Tower out of mashed potatoes in *Close Encounters*. But today there are just a couple of gentle hills. My seconds don't cover the plate. I skip thirds. I don't slip into the kitchen late at night for a turkey sandwich and leftover whatever au gratin. This is progress.

After a couple dark months, Alix and I are starting to feel the sun. My bosses at ESPN fought for me, and my contract got renewed. A stable check is a rare thing in journalism these days. Even better, I get to keep working with people I like. That's never a guarantee in any job. Alix is also starting to pick up more coaching clients. We have a lot to be thankful for.

On the road, I've started listening to podcasts. My favorite one is hosted by Brian Koppelman, who cowrote the poker movie *Rounders* and the Showtime series *Billions*, among many other things. Koppelman interviews other screenwriters, musicians, authors, self-help gurus—he loves to talk about the creative process, and how to give yourself permission to be special. One day his guest was his wife, Amy, a gifted novelist. She said something that made me pull over and write it down: *Your inner voice is telling you what you need to be. Sometimes it's whispering, sometimes it's shouting. Listen.*

It hits me hard because I realize that kind voice has always been in there, encouraging me to change my life. But only now is it starting to drown out USUCK-FM.

After Thanksgiving, our drive back home from Tennessee is 230 miles through the mountains—five hours if we stop a couple times. I used to mark every regular route we take by what we can eat on the way. My favorite stop on this trip is Bridges Barbecue Lodge in Shelby, North Carolina. Bridges, which is forty-five minutes from our house, is the second-best barbecue place in the world. (The best barbecue place in the world is Lexington Barbecue, about an hour from our house in the other direction.) We've stopped at Bridges countless times for chopped pork and fries and hush puppies. One time, traveling alone, I got a second order of hush puppies to go. It didn't last three red lights.

Whether I was hungry or not never used to matter. But this time we drive on past even though I think I feel my car jerk toward the parking lot out of reflex. By the time we get to Charlotte, the hunger has kicked in. We stop at a pizza place. My friend Michael Schur once said that when he eats two slices of pizza, he feels full and happy. When he eats four, he feels sick. He always eats four. I usually eat five or six. Tonight I eat three. We box up the rest and go home.

Weight on October 31: 439

Weight on November 30: 437

For the month: -2

For the year: -23

Twelve

DECEMBER/LIFE'S WORK

BRENDA'S PEANUT BUTTER LOGS

1 box 4x confectioners' sugar

1 cup shredded coconut

1 cup graham cracker crumbs

1 teaspoon vanilla

1 cup peanut butter

1 cup melted butter

1 cup pecans, chopped finely

Coating:

1 12-ounce package chocolate chips

½ block paraffin wax

Mix sugar, coconut, graham crackers, vanilla, and peanut butter. Add butter and pecans.

(You can now roll mixture into logs and quick-freeze on baking sheet, then place in freezer bags until ready to coat.)

Melt chocolate chips and paraffin together.

Dip frozen logs (using toothpicks) into chocolate mixture. Place on wax paper. As logs cool, chocolate will harden.

Makes about 50

Alix and I went back and forth over the peanut butter logs. We didn't know whether to make them or not. We wondered if they would soothe the wounds, or tear them back open.

My family doesn't have a lot of Christmas traditions. We open presents on whatever day everybody can get together. Mama has always had an artificial tree. The ornaments are whatever's on sale at Kmart. My old roommate Clint Engel had real tinsel, passed down through generations of his family, that he placed on the Christmas tree one strand at a time. I watched him in wonder and envy. My family had nothing like that. Except for Brenda's peanut butter logs.

Nobody remembers exactly when she started making them, or where the recipe came from. We've had them at Christmas for as long as I can remember. Every year Brenda and Mama would coat them together, getting chocolate all over their hands and the stove. They'd pack the logs in cookie tins. We'd get them out after the big Christmas meal. If you wanted to take some home, you had to hide them. Otherwise they'd be gone by dark.

Every year Mama fusses at Ronald for calling them "turds," but he's right—they look like the goose poop Fred used to eat. But they taste like Reese's cups, only a thousand times better. When I bite into one I see Brenda sitting across the old kitchen table, winking and letting loose that cackle of joy that was hers alone, trademarked and certified.

Every year we told the story about the time Brenda made dozens of uncoated logs in advance, planning to dip them in chocolate just before Christmas. She stashed them in the big freezer on their porch. Ed would walk by on the way to his shop and grab one now and then. There were a lot of now and thens. When Brenda went to the freezer just before Christmas, there were only two or three logs left. You might say she was slightly displeased. Later on she would laugh about it and tell the story herself, and we'd sympathize with her, but we'd also sympathize with Ed. You can't walk by a peanut butter log, even an unfinished one, without it calling your name.

I don't know what to do with that story now that Brenda's gone.

When she died last Christmas Eve, it wrecked us. We turned off the icicle lights and put on our funeral clothes. Now, a year later, it still feels like she just went down to the store. She'll be home any minute. Let's wait until she gets back.

Years ago, I wrote down Brenda's recipe on an index card. This year, Alix found it in our recipe box. We eventually decided to make some and take them to the family as a Christmas surprise. I was worried about two things with this plan: One, we might ruin Christmas. Two, I might eat all the logs before we get to Georgia.

That's the kind of thing the old me would have done.

.   .   .

It's a new morning. I get up and pee. I don't check Twitter. I put on some clothes and my New Balance sneakers. I'm walking before my mind catches up to what's going on. I do the same loop most of the time: down to the end of our street, across one block to the parallel street, back up that street, back across to our house. It's right at a mile. I read the paper and eat breakfast—bran flakes, 1 percent milk, a banana if we've got some, ice water. I sit down at my desk. There's a notebook with a to-do list for the week, and another notebook with a grid blocking out my day. I set a timer for forty-five minutes. I work until the timer goes off and take a fifteen-minute break. Rinse, repeat.

That's how it goes when everything works.

Lots of days, something goes sideways. I sleep too late. I decide it's crucial to know what people are saying on social media at 7:30 in the morning. I talk myself out of walking. I talk myself into a breakfast PB&J. I read a vitally important story about SEC football recruiting. I follow a forty-five-minute shift with a two-hour nap.

I am still adjusting to the idea of being an adult.

This, in the end, is what it's about for me. To control my weight, to get in shape, to become the person I'm supposed to be, I have to shake the habits that have clung to me since I was a kid. Chances are you've heard the lines from I Corinthians, probably at a wedding: *When I was a child, I spoke as a child, I understood as a child, I thought as a child; but when I became a man, I put away childish things.* I've never quite believed in that verse. I don't want to put away the child inside me. But I can't let him run the house, either. And that's what he's been doing my whole life.

Years ago I saw the author Tom Wolfe speak. His novels tend to be about people who let their lives get way out of hand. In his speech, he criticized the "loose life" he saw so many people trying to get away with—shaky morals, bad habits, ready-made excuses. Problem was, the loose life sounded great to me. That's what I'd always hoped for—a life I could live however I wanted without any real consequences. I didn't want to murder or pillage or cheat on my wife. I didn't mind working because I loved to write. But otherwise I craved a Big Lebowski life. Drift along, hang out with friends, keep a cocktail in hand at all times. Skip the White Russians. Give me bourbon over ice.

The loosest life I wanted was with food, because food has given me more pleasure than anything else. That doesn't mean I like food more than sex. It just means I haven't had sex three (or four or five) times a day for fifty-one years. That's Hugh Hefner. I've eaten too much of too many bad things for the cheap thrill of it, trying to stay one step ahead of paying the price, like a grifter kiting checks. I knew how much it would cost me later. But I craved that moment of joy now.

That's the way a child thinks.

Alix and I have started using the word *adulting*. When we wash the supper dishes right away instead of waiting until midnight, we're adulting. When we file away papers instead of letting them pile up in a stack, we're adulting. I've come to realize that adulting is the only way I can beat my addiction to food.

The other day I wrote up a little guide to my adulthood:

- I have to lose weight to have a longer, healthier, more meaningful life.
- I have to do it in a way I can live with tomorrow and tomorrow and tomorrow.
- I have to find other sources of joy and solace, especially in hard times.
- I have to accept delayed gratification.
- I have to mute the self-hating voice in my head.
- I have to believe that I'm worth saving.
- I have to do all this not just for myself, but for the people who love me.

All this means work. It means following the Three-Step Diet every day, measuring what I'm eating and what I'm burning. It means quitting fast food and convenience-store crap. It means not just turning off USUCK-FM, but taking the boom box outside and smashing that fucker with a sledgehammer. It means being more professional in my job and more structured in my life so I'm less stressed and less likely to binge. It means being honest with the people I love, and honest with myself.

I've resisted those things all these years because it felt like so much work. It *is* work. But the loose life—the life that looked like so much fun—turned out to be a fraud. It got me to 460 pounds. It made me an actuarial disaster. It threatens my life. It limits me more than a disciplined life ever could.

My childhood didn't give me a great start. I was a sedentary child who grew up on the normal Southern diet for people who stayed on their feet all day. I learned to love all those calories as friends when I didn't have many. As I got older, my choices made things a whole lot worse. I gravitated to salt, sugar, and fat (and the fourth element: alcohol). I never cared enough about myself to think it mattered. My approach to life sent me off in the wrong direction, and it took me forever to turn around and head back. I don't know how close I got to falling off the cliff. It's foggy out there. I could slip and fall. All I know is that I'm finally walking away from the edge.

I'm still stumbling around trying to answer that question those assholes asked me at that party twenty-five years ago: *Tommy, why are you so fat?* But here's something I've come to believe: The answer doesn't matter as much as the action. You can't wait until you're ready. Nobody's ever ready. I wish I had more time to loll around in my loose life. But it's time to tighten up.

We make it to Georgia with the same number of peanut butter logs we left with. We celebrate Christmas on the day after Christmas because that's when all the family can get together. Nineteen of us crowd into Mama's little living room and kitchen. We say grace before supper. Mama cries a little and says how much she misses Brenda. We have a quiet moment in her name. Amen.

Ham and KFC, boiled shrimp and sausage balls, field peas and potato salad, squash casserole and coleslaw. Sliced tomatoes and cucumbers and green onions and beets. Red velvet cake, pound cake, Hershey's kiss cookies, apple pie. There is enough for an army battalion. But we are professionals. We transfer the food from the plates to our bellies with speed and precision and love. I try not to pile it up, but the sausage balls are my weakness. As I reach for another, I can hear my Fitbit weep.

People start to move in on the desserts and so Alix and I unveil our hidden stash of peanut butter logs. It turns out to be a nice moment. Normally we'd all just dive in. But now we take a little time to remember. Ed, Brenda's husband, is not much for showing his feelings in public. He just takes out a log and smiles: "I didn't think I'd see one of these this year."

I don't know what the others think when they eat theirs, but I give thanks for Brenda, and Fred, and my job, and my family, and all the things that got me here, good and bad.

Food will never be just a quick, cheap pleasure for me. Sometimes it's a path back to the best moments of my life with the people I love. Maybe I kept eating because I kept trying to find those moments. Only now do I realize they can be small and sacred. A peanut butter log and a sip of sweet tea wouldn't pass for a church Communion. But here, now, it's enough.

Most years, over the five or six days around Christmas, I'd eat twenty-five or thirty peanut butter logs.

This year I have four and a half.

Weight on November 30: 437
Weight on December 31: 435

For the month: -2

For the year: -25

Twenty-five pounds in a year might not sound like much to you. A lot of diet plans promise that in a month. By now you know what I think of those diet plans. Still, the numbers get stuck in our heads. We see the stories on the cover of *People*, all those women who lost 150 pounds in a year. Judged by that standard, you might think twenty-five pounds barely matter. Let me tell you what those twenty-five pounds mean to me.

I've never lost twenty-five pounds in a year. I might have been down twenty-five pounds at some point, but I always gained it all back and then some. Now, for the first time in my life, keeping the weight off feels sustainable. I still have a cheeseburger every once in a while. But now it's two or three a month instead of two or three a day.

My cholesterol and blood pressure were high enough that Dr. Hudson thought about putting me on medication. Now they're back to normal levels. The only pills I take every day are vitamins.

My right Achilles used to hurt like hell every morning. It hasn't flared up in months. I used to wake up with headaches from sleeping so poorly. That almost never happens now.

I'm down a size across the board. I threw out my size sixty jeans once the size fifty-eights fit for a month. Now the new jeans are loose. My belt is on its last hole. My shirts are down from 6X to 5X.

I'm substituting other rewards for food. I buy a new book when

I hit a goal. I comb the racks at Lunchbox Records, down the street from our house. Sometimes I just drive around Charlotte for a couple hours. One of my favorite places in town is the overlook park near the airport. It's next to a couple of runways so I can watch the planes take off and land. There's a mesmerizing rhythm to it. There's also a Wendy's not far away. I used to stop by for a double cheeseburger combo before I went to the park. The last couple times, I've had a glass of ice water I brought from the house.

Walking is easier. Our house is three blocks from a main drag with a bank, library, post office, grocery store, lots of restaurants and bars, and four tattoo parlors. The main reason we chose our house was so we could walk places. I'm ashamed to say how many times I've driven those three blocks to meet somebody for lunch. But lately I've been walking down there. Alix noticed that I'm not griping as much when we walk. I'm never going to be a guy who wanders the world on foot. My goals are more modest. I'd like to walk a 10K sometime. Maybe walk uptown (about three miles), see a ball game or something, and walk back. There's a bridge on the way where photographers line up at night to take pictures of the Charlotte skyline. I've never walked across that bridge. I've been wondering if my iPhone camera could get a good shot.

All this happened in one of the roughest years I can remember. Fred died near the end. Alix left her job and I nearly lost mine. Brenda's death pressed down on our family like cinder blocks. Most years I would've come out the other end fatter than when I started. But I tried to honor my sister, and value my family and friends. Most of all, I came to believe I was someone worth saving.

Go to the gym and pick up a twenty-five-pound dumbbell, or go to the hardware store and lift a twenty-five-pound bag of mulch. Hold it for a while, let it be part of you. Think about the load you have to carry. Now set it down and walk away. That's what I did this year.

So that twenty-five pounds means a lot to me.

Of course I have to lose more. I've tried not to make long-term goals. But the truth is that I have one. I want to get down to 230 pounds. That might still be overweight by medical standards, but if I get to 230, I'll be half the man I was. I'm hoping to get there in four or five years. But I'm not going to worry about when as much as how. I'm boarding up the doors behind me. I don't plan on going back.

I'll always struggle with food. That hog is a part of me, as fundamental as bone and blood. But the thing about getting in shape is that you develop untapped strength, and not just in your muscles. It turns out I'm a better fighter than I thought.

My morning ritual used to be a long naked look in the mirror and a scoop of self-hate before breakfast. Now I see a different man. And the morning routine has a different spin.

Wake up.

Still fat.

Well, hell.

OK, then.

Back to work.

EPILOGUE

NEW YEAR'S DAY, 2017

My 2016 in six words: *Gave up fast food for Lent.*

This was back in February. On Fat Tuesday, the day of feasting, I got Wendy's one last time for lunch. On Ash Wednesday we went to the evening service at our church, and I made a silent vow that I was done with all the fast-food chains—anyplace with a drive-through, ketchup packets, and food that comes in a bag. Since that day I have stayed away from McDonald's and Taco Bell and KFC and their kin. There has been one exception: the day I took my mom to the doctor, and she decided on the way home that she wanted biscuits at Hardee's. When your mama wants biscuits at Hardee's, you get biscuits at Hardee's. I trust that God gave me a pass.

That was March 9. I stuck the receipt in my billfold. For years I did that every time I ate some terrible fast-food meal, swearing every time that it would be the last one. Again and again I made myself a liar. But that Hardee's receipt has stayed in my billfold for 298 days and counting. The ink is so faded, I can barely see what I ate.

Since Lent I have snacked on potato chips a few times, but I haven't once emptied a family-sized bag. I have indulged in a Little Debbie once or twice, but I haven't even glanced at a whole box. The hardest thing to kick has been sweet tea. I am a lifelong Southerner. Sweet tea is our blood type. So I am giving myself a gradual transfusion of unsweet tea and Coke Zero and water. So far, my body has not rejected these foreign substances.

I've had cravings, sure. One day in September I drove from Charlotte to Harlan, Kentucky, for a story. I got there late and hungry. I drove down the main drag and all the bright lights were temptations: Arby's, Taco Bell, Pizza Hut, my former sweetheart Wendy. I just about gave in. Then I found a Food City supermarket that was open until midnight. I got a turkey sandwich from the deli and a Diet Coke. I'm not going to pretend it was as good as a Quarter Pounder, but when I got back home I was able to put an X in that box on the calendar where I am marking the days I have held to my pledge. The calendar is now a big unbroken string of X's, and each one of those is its own jolt of pleasure.

The next day in Kentucky, I got bit by a dog. It wasn't that bad a bite, and the dog had its shots. I went home with a scar and a story.

I've started thinking about my life as a fat man the same way. I've got scars, and I've got stories. Now I just have to get home.

. . .

These days my pants are falling off for the right reason. They used to fall off because my gut was so big that it pushed my waistband down to my knees. Now they fall off because the waistband is too big. I have gone from a tight size sixty to a loose fifty-six. This is a new feeling, buying smaller clothes. My hand has always gone to the far end of the rack. Now I have to pull it back toward the middle.

A couple months ago I was in Walmart, and on the way out I walked by a stack of six-dollar sweatshirts. They went up to 4X. I thought *what the hell*, and took one home, and damn if it doesn't fit. Not counting socks, that's the first piece of clothing I remember getting from a regular store since those childhood husky jeans at Sears.

When I rent a car now, I don't have to try out three or four until I find one where the seat belt buckles. When I go to the movies, I don't have to flip up the armrest between the seats. My one suit—the suit I thought I'd be buried in—hangs on me now like the one David Byrne wore in *Stop Making Sense*. It's going to Goodwill as soon as I buy a new one.

I have performed a magical anti-aging trick: I've erased some of the worry lines around Alix's eyes. When we go out to eat, and I skip the burger for grilled chicken, she smiles and says: "What have you done with my husband?" When she hugs me now, her arms go all the way around me. To feel her fingertips touch at the small of my back is a pleasure no meal can match.

Let me be clear: I am still a sinner. There is a Dairy Queen five blocks from our house, and sometimes on a summer night I will dive into a Blizzard with Oreos. If we're back home in Georgia, and

Mama is cooking, I'm having ham and lima beans and cornbread, and then I'm having a nap. Her living room has a couch that reclines, plus a regular recliner. It's a docking station for food comas.

But eating until I pass out is a rare thing now. When it comes to food I am finally growing up, and grown people do things in moderation.

It will never be easy. Right now, for example, I am thinking about chocolate chips. Alix uses them for baking and always keeps a stash around the house. She hides them from me for my own good. The other day, looking for something in the back of the freezer, I found them. I haven't touched them yet. But I can taste them in my mind, right out of the freezer bag, warming in my mouth until they melt together. Those sensations will roll around in my head as long as I have an imagination. The difference is, moment by moment, day by day, I have started to detach the thinking from the doing.

Why has it worked this time when it never worked before? Maybe because this time I decided to change in a slow and steady way that I might be able to sustain. Maybe because I knew I would be writing a book about life as a fat man, and I wanted to show by the end that I had a chance to be something else.

Most of all, though, Brenda's death shook me. My only sister died a terrible death from something directly connected to her weight. I saw what it did to the rest of us for her to leave so soon. I don't want to put my family through that again. I want all the time I can get with the people I love.

It could be that I have started too late, that I've done damage to my body that can't be fixed. My right knee still wobbles and grinds, and I'll have to get it replaced someday. My calves are still rust-colored from the veins that can't push the blood up high enough. Every time a pocket of gas forms in my chest, I have the same panicked thought—*heart attack*—before I belch it out. There could be a clot in one of my arteries, a time bomb in my liver, a weak spot in my small intestine, a debt that has yet to come due.

It was a stressful work year. This time around, when my contract came up, ESPN really did let me go—along with a bunch of other people. That was my most stable writing gig. But other assignments filled the space, and even though it was more of a scramble, I always had a couple stories going. Alix was scrambling, too, trying to get her coaching business fully launched. But our life felt more peaceful once my weight wasn't a constant worry. Those normal daily stresses didn't seem to matter as much as they used to.

What matters to me right now—even more than losing weight—is that I'm trying. I never tried this hard before. I thought it was hopeless because I thought I was hopeless. I used to worry about lying to myself about being able to stick to a diet and get in shape. Now I see I told myself a bigger lie: that I wasn't worth the trouble.

I am still a fat man. I will probably always be one in my head, even if I shed every pound I want to lose. But I know for sure now that there is another man inside me. And I'm no longer scared to meet him.

For the first part of the year I weigh in at the YMCA, which has a scale that goes up to five hundred pounds. In the summer, on a trip to Costco, I buy a scale for our house—the first scale I've ever bought. It tops out at four hundred. The first few times I step on, the digital readout says ERROR.

On the last day of August, I step on, and the numbers roll around like a slot machine. When they stop, and I look down, the readout says 399. (In the interest of full disclosure, it says 399.5, but you bet your ass I'm rounding down.)

When was the last time my weight started with a three? Before I was married, for sure. Probably not since I lived in Augusta more than thirty years ago.

I keep looking at the number. I want to dance and I want to cry.

Around the corner from the scale, out in the hall, there's an old family photo Alix restored for me for Christmas one year. It's at a boat landing on the Altamaha River, where my family caught all those sweet catfish when I was growing up. This photo is not on a fishing day—it's a special trip. My dad is wearing a dress shirt and khakis. Brenda, a teenager, is smiling next to him. And in my dad's lap, there I am: a baby, eyes closed, bald as a butter bean.

In that moment, I could have turned out to be anything. I didn't have to be a kid who snuck cheese out of the refrigerator, a teenager who stole sandwiches at school, a college kid who drank way too much beer, a young man who quit running and jumping, a middle-aged guy who caused pain and worry for the people who loved him. I could have been better. I want to reach back into that photo and tell that little baby to live a different life. But as my friend Thomas Lake once wrote: *Time is a dark blue river, and it rolls one way.*

Instead I think about Daddy and Brenda, both so happy in that picture. I'm skeptical that our loved ones look down at us from heaven. But sometimes you believe what you need to believe.

I close my eyes and say with my mind:

I miss you two.

I wish you were here.

I'm sorry it took me so long to lose weight.

I'm finally doing it.

I hope you can see.

I don't know how much guilt weighs. Guilt and shame are the hardest weight to shed. But that morning I feel some of it lift off of me.

I spend New Year's Eve in Washington, D.C., working on a story about a civil-rights preacher named Reverend William Barber. He leads rallies all over the country, telling young activists not to give up even when things look their worst. One of the points he makes in every sermon is that the Montgomery bus boycott, which started when Rosa Parks refused to give up her seat, lasted 381 days. It's a simple message: Put in the work every day, stick to the plan, and monumental things can happen.

In between interviews I stroll around the city, walking longer and lighter than I used to. Never once do I get tired. I call home and tell Alix I love her, and I'll see her in the New Year. At the end of the day I look over my work, check my Fitbit, write down what I ate, and fall into an easy sleep.

This all started with a dream about a hog. Its attack was relentless. It stood for all my weaknesses, all my fears, all my self-hatred, everything that was causing me to kill myself one combo meal at a time. We all have a beast in us somewhere. Yours might be shoplifting or gossip or drugs. Mine is food. I can't kill the hog, but maybe I can tame it. It respects order and effort. For the first time in my life, it's curled up in the corner peacefully. I don't dream about it anymore. I've got different dreams now.

Weight on December 31, 2015: 435

Weight on January 1, 2017: 386

For the year 2016: -49

Overall (2015 and 2016): -74

P.S.

Weight on January 1, 2017: 386

Weight on Thanksgiving 2017: 375

For the year: -11

Overall (2015–2017): -85

Acknowledgments

This is going to be like at the Oscars where the winner of some minor category gets up and talks for so long the orchestra starts playing that "get the hell off the stage" music. I don't care. There are so many people to thank.

First off, some teachers: Lillian Williams at Jane Macon Middle School; Brenda Hunt, Wayne Ervin, and James Holt at Brunswick High School; and Conrad Fink at the University of Georgia. All of them showed me a bigger world, and handed me maps to get there.

Next, some editors: James Folker at the *Augusta Chronicle*; Trisha O'Connor, John Bordsen, John Drescher, Gary Schwab, Cheryl Carpenter, Cindy Montgomery, and Mike Gordon at the *Charlotte Observer*; Chris Stone at *Sports Illustrated*; Jena Janovy at *ESPN the Magazine* and ESPN.com; Megan Greenwell, then at *Esquire*, now at *Deadspin*; and many others I will regret not mentioning the moment this book comes out. My butt has also been saved a million times over by copyeditors, especially Beryl Adcock and

Roger Mikeal at the *Observer*. Repeat after me from the scripture: Everybody needs an editor.

I want to set aside a paragraph for two special editors. Frank Barrows at the *Observer* chose me to be the local columnist—the most important thing that ever happened in my career—and stood by me when I almost blew the whole thing. I still look to him for wisdom and guidance. Jay Lovinger at ESPN taught me more just by talking on the phone than any other editor ever has with a pen or a delete key. He's a guru I'd climb a mountain for.

I dug back through old emails and found my first exchange with my agent, Sloan Harris. It was in 2006. This book is coming out in 2019. Sloan is a patient man. He spent years gently rejecting dozens of my terrible ideas and shaping a few others that were worth a discussion but not quite a book. When we hit on this idea, he waited even longer because I was afraid to write it. Then, when I was finally ready, he sold the thing in what felt like ten seconds. Thank you, sir. I wish we could go to Anderson's and celebrate this.

Jofie Ferrari-Adler at Simon & Schuster did his most important work as the editor of this book before I wrote a word of it. When Sloan was shopping it around to publishers, Jofie called me to say how much he loved the idea and that he would be thrilled to make the book the best that it could be. By the end of the call, I would've bought a time-share in a condo from him. He made the book better every time he touched it and was a joy to work with every step of the way.

There are so many people I've never even met at Simon & Schuster who did such great work on this book. Julianna Haubner and

Kristen Lemire kept the trains running. Jessica Chin, the copyediting manager, and Marla Jea, the copyeditor, handled literally thousands of changes to the manuscript. Jamie Keenan designed the jacket, Ruth Lee-Mui designed the interior, and Kate Barrett handled corrections in desktop. Nicole Hines is handling the marketing and Maddie Schmitz is doing publicity. Please let me know what gifts y'all want from the Carolinas. We have multiple varieties of barbecue sauce.

A few of many, many friends: Perry Beard from back home in Brunswick; David Duclos, Zane Vanhook, Jon Bauer, Kim Clemons, and Ellen Lord from UGA; Clint Engel, John Prince, and Tim Richardson from Augusta; Ann Helms, Kathi Purvis, Doug Miller, Diane Suchetka, Dan Huntley, Ken Garfield, Jim Walser, and a million others from the *Charlotte Observer*; my fellow Bad Niemans from the 2008–09 Nieman Fellowship, especially Rosita Boland and Chris Vognar, who gave feedback on an early draft, and curator Bob Giles, who brought us all together; Greg Collard, Ju-Don Marshall, Nick de la Canal, Lisa Worf, Joe O'Connor, and everybody else I'm getting to know at WFAE; and Chris Jones, Mike Schur, Kevin Van Valkenburg, Chuck Culpepper, Michael Kruse, Ben Montgomery, Mike Graff, Tony Rehagen, Thomas Lake, Greg Lacour, Lisa Rab, Gavin Edwards, Lisa Pollak, Jeremy Markovich, Jonathan Abrams, and so many others from out in the writing world. Spouses, too.

Joe Posnanski did it all before me—wrote a column, worked for magazines, blogged, podcasted, wrote books. Most of what I've learned about these things, I've learned from watching him. We threw a baseball around in his apartment parking lot nearly thirty years ago, two bureau reporters in Rock Hill, South Carolina, wondering if we'd ever make it to our version of the bigs. I think we got there. Thanks for the advice and the friendship and the many, many three-hour lunches.

My family is everything. I couldn't have made it here without my brother, Ronald Bennett, his wife, Neca, and their children, Gina and Brett; my late sister, Brenda Williams, her husband, Ed, and their children Alison, Alisha, and Jerod; my mother-in-law, Joann Felsing, and her children, Rich and Christie; and all the cousins and uncles and aunts dotting every corner of the South and beyond. Thanks for supporting me even when some of you didn't quite understand what I do for a living. Sometimes I don't understand it either.

As I was in the final stretch of writing this book, three of the people who meant the most to me died in a span of five months. I'll never be able to say enough, here or anywhere, about Virgil Ryals, my best friend; Dick Felsing, my father-in-law; and especially Virginia Tomlinson, my mom, who died in January 2018 after a long illness. I hope you see in these pages how much I loved her. She lived long enough to see an early version of the book. She thought it was good except for the cussing.

I can't mention my mom without mentioning my dad, L.M. Tomlinson (1915–1990). See you in my dreams, Daddy.

The orchestra has been playing for a while now, the broadcast has cut to commercial, but I'm not leaving until I say this: Marrying Alix Felsing is the greatest thing that ever happened to me, or ever will. You know from reading the book how much I have put her through. She has handled it all with strength and humor and grace. Every day I think I love her to full capacity, but the next day I love her more. It seems impossible. But with Alix, nothing is.

About the Author

TOMMY TOMLINSON spent twenty-three years as a reporter and columnist for the *Charlotte Observer*, where he was a finalist for the 2005 Pulitzer Prize in commentary. He has written for publications including *ESPN The Magazine*, *Esquire*, *Sports Illustrated*, and *Garden & Gun*. His stories have been chosen twice for the Best American Sports Writing series. He now hosts the podcast *SouthBound* from WFAE, Charlotte's NPR news station. He lives in Charlotte with his wife, Alix Felsing.